Reiki and the
Healing Buddha

By Maureen J. Kelly

LOTUS
PRESS

P.O. Box 325
Twin Lakes, WI 53181

2nd Printing 2001
Library of Congress Cataloging-in-Publication Data
Kelly, Maureen
Reiki and the Healing Buddha
ISBN: 0-914955-92-6
1. Subject   I. Title
Library of Congress Control Number   00-090029

Published By:
Lotus Press
P.O. Box 325
Twin Lakes, Wisconsin 53181
Web: www.lotuspress.com
e-mail: lotuspress@lotuspress.com

ACKNOWLEDGEMENTS

I am grateful to Raoul Birnbaum for writing the book The Healing Buddha and Alex Wayman and F D Lessing for their studies of the Healing Buddha, the Seven Healing Buddhas and Tantric Buddhism. My thanks go to the authors whose books are listed in the Bibliography of this book for writing a phrase, sentence, paragraph or more in their books which enabled me to discover more about Reiki, and also to those scholars who translated Buddhist texts and sutras into English, the only language I can read.

I acknowledge and honour my Reiki lineage. Mikao Usui for rediscovering Reiki, for bringing it out of the Buddhist monastery and making it available to everyone. Chujiro Hayashi for his contribution to Reiki and for allowing Hawayo Takata to become a Reiki Master. Hawayo Takata for bringing Reiki to the west.

THE PAST BUDDHAS OF REIKI
Mikao Usui
Chujiro Hayashi
Hawayo Takata

First Degree	Second Degree	Third Degree
Barbara Ray	Phyllis Furumoto	Iris Ishikura
John Latz	Bobbe Free	Arthur Robertson
Clarity Martin	Maureen Kelly	DianeMcCumber MarleneSchilke
Carrlyn Harring		William Lee Rand
Victoria Sinclair		Barbara Pillsbury
Maureen Kelly		Maureen Kelly

iii

CONTENTS

INTRODUCTION

A well-known American Reiki Master once told me that she had "gone past Reiki". Reiki, as it is presently taught, lacks the depth and complexity that the human mind likes. After several years at master level a Reiki practitioner can feel as though they have come to a dead end. When this happens it becomes necessary to reach back into the rich and intricate heritage from which Reiki has come for greater depth and understanding.

As I progressed through the Reiki degrees I found myself searching for more. The feeling of "Is this all?" would not go away. It led me to take several Second Degree Advanced classes with Reiki Master Randall Hayward, who had been researching Reiki for several years, and Margaret Underwood who had done her Reiki Master training with Randall. During one class a desire was triggered within me to do my own research into the Reiki symbols. Although my search began with the Reiki symbols, it eventually widened to encompass the whole Reiki system leading me to a new understanding of the Reiki Story and to Reiki's relationship to Buddhism and in particular to the Healing Buddha.

The journey has been one of discovery of both myself and of Reiki. The more I have learned about Reiki the more amazed I have been about Reiki and the more I have come to love and appreciate this wondrous energy that we call Reiki. For me it has become more understandable while remaining one of the great mysteries of our times.

The sacredness of the Reiki symbols has, I believe, never really been understood nor truly acknowledged within Reiki.

This book is my attempt to explain why these symbols are sacred as well as point out the symbolism of the Reiki Story, and to bring to Reiki practitioners a deeper understanding of both. The Reiki symbols have appeared in other books with, I believe, inadequate or incorrect information about them. Unfortunately those books, as the only published records of the Reiki symbols, have become written authorities on the symbols. This book is also my attempt to "set the records straight" concerning Reiki and its symbols. Because of the numbers of Reiki practitioners and masters in the world today the only way to reach the majority is by the written word rather than the traditional oral communication which is the normal practice of Reiki.

This book has been primarily written for those who have already attended Reiki classes and had the energy we know as Reiki activated within them. The reader cannot and will not become a Reiki practitioner or master simply by reading this book. By far the most important element of the Reiki system is the initiation ritual which is performed by the Reiki Master during a Reiki class. This ritual activates the chakras and attunes students' life force to the creative healing power of the universe so that they can channel the Universal Life Force Energy (Reiki) through their hands easily, whenever they place their hands on themselves or someone else. To my knowledge the Reiki initiation is unique. It may be similar to the initiation Jesus Christ gave his disciples so they could heal with their hands as He did, which is now lost to Christianity. Its nearest counterpart today is the "empowerments" or consecrations administered by Buddhist monks.

It is my hope that this book will also help those who translate the sacred and spiritual writings of Asia to take seriously such things as symbols, initiations, life force and healing energies for it is my experience that they are not just

2

words. For me Reiki is evidence that symbols, initiations and life force energy are dynamic and effective.

My respect for Mikao Usui, who rediscovered the method of healing known as Reiki, has increased enormously. How did he find his way through the sutras, decipher their meanings and become initiated to the energy itself? I found it a slow, painstaking struggle to wade through the Buddhist writings, and I knew about Reiki before I started, he didn't. The other thing which amazes me about Mikao Usui is that he took Reiki out of Buddhism and made it available to everyone.

Chapter 1

WHAT IS REIKI?

The word Reiki is the result of combining the Japanese words Rei and Ki. The Japanese dictionary usually allocates the idea of spirit or ghost to the word Rei, and life force energy to the word Ki. Mrs Takata gave the meaning of Reiki as Universal Life Force Energy, with Rei meaning Universal and Ki meaning Life Force Energy. She likened Reiki to a broadcast from a radio station and Duff Cady in his article *Reiki Returns to Hawayo Takata's House* discovered that Mrs Takata referred to Reiki treatments as "Shortwave Treatments."

Explaining exactly what Reiki is and where it comes from is often very hard to do. Consequently there are many explanations. The following is my explanation.

Rei–Universal/Spiritual Energy

Reiki is most often described as a light vibration or energy, and Reiki practitioners are said to "channel" it from the universe. Our planet is bombarded with vibrational waves and particles from the sun and from suns much further away, which we refer to as stars. The most obvious energy we receive from the sun is sunlight. Our eyes have developed to use this light to see, and especially to see colours. However, we do not see the whole range of rays contained within sunlight; known as the "electromagnetic light spectrum". This spectrum contains visible light, radio waves, shortwaves, microwaves, x-rays, infra-red, ultra-violet, gamma rays and cosmic rays and probably rays or waves which have not yet been discovered. This electromagnetic spectrum of light bombards earth day and night.

It is my belief that the Rei of Reiki is one of the rays of the light spectrum which has yet to be discovered by scientists. My experience with using crystals for healing has led me to believe that our brain has the ability to filter out or accept and use very fine vibrations which cannot be seen or heard. Although we can use Reiki at any time of the day or night a number of Reiki practitioners have commented to me that Reiki appears to be stronger when they do a Reiki treatment outside in sunlight or during the summer months.

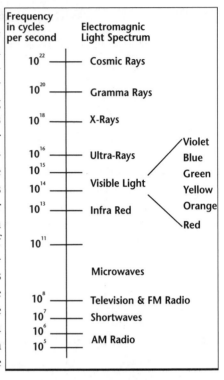

Frequency in cycles per second	Electromagnic Light Spectrum
10^{22}	Cosmic Rays
10^{20}	Gramma Rays
10^{18}	X-Rays
10^{16}	Ultra-Rays
10^{15}	
10^{14}	Visible Light
10^{13}	Infra Red
10^{11}	
	Microwaves
10^{8}	Television & FM Radio
10^{7}	Shortwaves
10^{6}	
10^{5}	AM Radio

Visible Light colours: Violet, Blue, Green, Yellow, Orange, Red

I believe that the Rei of Reiki is absorbed from the light spectrum through our eyes; the need for the practitioner to close their eyes during a Reiki treatment would indicate that this absorption also takes place through our third eye which can process light while we are sleeping.

The use of television, microwaves, shortwaves and radiowaves indicates that information can be sent via the light spectrum. We collect information about our world through visible light—because of visible light we see the shapes and colours of our world. Therefore it is not beyond belief that

1. What is Reiki?

the Rei of Reiki can also provide us with information and many Reiki practitioners have the experience of receiving profound and relevant information during Reiki treatments.

Our brainwaves and thought waves can align with the vibrational waves of the light spectrum and therefore we can use thoughts/intents to enhance and assist a Reiki treatment.

In *The Healing Buddha* by Raoul Birnbaum, lapis lazuli, the gem stone which is strongly associated with the Healing Buddha who is referred to as Lapis Lazuli Radiance, is described by the monk Hui-in (788-810) as being a divine substance created in the celestial realm—not stone created by fire or smelted by men; which leads me to believe lapis lazuli is a symbol for the Rei of Reiki, and that myrobalan (the healing herb usually held by the Healing Buddha) is the symbol for the life force energy (Ki).

Ki –Life Force Energy

Life force energy is known in many cultures around the world and has many names. The ones we are most familiar with today are probably India's Prana and China's Chi (or Qi) which is equivalent to Japan's Ki. Two popular Chinese methods of working with the life force energy are Tai Chi and Qi Kong. They both have exercises for developing, maintaining, enhancing and manipulating the life force energy within a person.

Life force energy is the energy which maintains life within humans and other living beings. Therefore if there is no life force energy there is no life. If we do not breathe, drink or eat eventually we will stop living, therefore the life force energy must come from what we breathe, drink and eat. In India prana is interpreted as breath and breathing.

I believe that the Ki of Reiki comes from the air we breathe, the water we drink and the food we eat. Air, water and food are the fuels which the body converts to energy. From both air and water we get oxygen, which the cells of our body and brain use constantly, and from food comes the calories which creates the energy we need to be active. Scientists have been able to discover which part of our brain works when we do something by looking for an increase of iron. It is iron in the blood which transports oxygen around the body. A high incidence of iron indicates oxygen is not being used. When a part of the brain is working it is unable to take in more oxygen and can only use the oxygen that is already stored in its cells. The same thing also happens when a muscle is working. Therefore when a part of the brain runs out of oxygen, you will get a headache. Likewise your muscles will ache when they lack oxygen. If the brain is deprived of oxygen you may even faint or lose consciousness. Yawning is one method the body uses to increase the intake of oxygen. Athletes train so their muscles utilise oxygen and calories better, enabling them to use their muscles for longer and longer periods of time.

By observing Reiki practitioners at Support Groups you will note that after doing two or three Reiki treatments they begin yawning or they develop a headache (usually across the forehead) and can feel quite sleepy, indicating that their brains may be short of oxygen. If a Reiki practitioner has eaten little or no food during the day they may feel faint while giving a Reiki treatment. After giving several Reiki treatments or after doing several attunements a Reiki practitioner can also feel quite hungry. Most Reiki teachers stress the importance for people giving and receiving Reiki to drink lots of water. The oxygen from water can be sent from the stomach to the brain quite quickly. Taking several deep breaths between treatments and having something to eat before a treatment also helps. Doing lots of Reiki treatments regularly on yourself or giving them to others is like an athlete training and is probably one of the major reasons why it has traditionally been important to spend time practicing Reiki between the Reiki degrees. You will be able to utilise the life force energy from air, water and food better and more efficiently, effectively enabling you to give Reiki for longer periods of time. This is particularly pertinent for Reiki Masters who give Reiki initiations to large groups of people. It takes time to build up this kind of stamina. Doing Tai Chi, Qi Kong, or swimming, jogging and other exercises will also help to increase your ability to use the life force energy more effectively.

Reiki, I believe, combines the vibrations of light waves (the spiritual energy of the universe) and the life force energy to enable the body to relax and heal, and the mind to become peaceful. Although there are other methods which utilise the life force energy, Reiki appears to be the only method which consistently, effortlessly and effectively enables us to use it with the spiritual energy or light waves of the universe.

Chapter 2

Symbols of Buddhism

Buddhism abounds with symbols and symbolism. There appears to be two kinds of Buddhist symbols which have the greatest relevance to Reiki; bija or seed symbols and mandalas. This is not to say that these are the only symbols which apply to Reiki. Because Reiki comes from Buddhism all symbols within Buddhism must have some relevance to Reiki. Mandalas and bijas are the most obvious to me at this time.

Bija or Seed Symbols

Bija means seed or essence. In Buddhism a bija is the seed or essence of an energetic force personified as either a Buddha or Bodhisattva. A bija is seen as the subtle body of that energy or deity. Bijas, as abstract symbols, connect at a high metaphysical level and therefore are considered to possess enormous power. Their most important purpose is to assist the worshipper to become "one" with a particular deity or energy.

The letters of the alphabet are not mere strokes drawn on paper, but powers vibrating with life; conscious sound-powers, symbols of cosmic power conceived as sound. Sound is identified with the power behind the cosmos. The conch shell symbolises the sounds of Buddha. Mandalas composed of letters of the Sanskrit alphabet represent the voice of Buddha.

The energetic forces of the universe can be symbolised in three ways—as a Buddha; as the symbol held by the Buddha; as a bija. Together these three types of symbols express the trinity of Heaven, Earth and Man (or Father, Mother, Child or King, Queen & Prince). There is a fourth level which represents going beyond the trinity to connection and integration with the cosmos. Ancient Buddhists, when asked to describe this level, would reply with silence because this level was, and still is, considered to be unexplainable.

Level 1
Physical
EARTH

Crescent Moon

Level 1 represents the form of the energy. It affects us at the levelwhich observes and is aware of the environment. At this level nature nourishes and sustains humanity. This is the level at which Feng Shui works.

Level 2
Mental/Emotional
MAN

Chandra
(Moon Buddha)

Level 2 is the personification of energy. It is available to us on our hidden subconscious and psychological levels. It is at this level that legends and myths work.

Level 3
Spiritual
HEAVEN

月

Kanji symbol
for Moon

Level 3 is the abstract level of the energy. It affects us on a deep spiritual level–the archetypal level. It is at this level that the four Reiki symbols work.

Level 4
Cosmic
NIRVANA

No Symbol

Level 4 has no forms or symbols and is known as emptiness, the void or Buddhahood. It is beyond symbols and forms and this level is believed to be reached during "Enlightenment".

All three symbols represent the same energy (Moon = benevolence) but are depicted in different ways at the different levels.

2. Symbols of Buddhism

The Mandala

There appear to be several types of mandalas used in Buddhism. One seems to be influenced by both the ancient ziggurats of Mesopotamia and the Ba Gua found in Feng Shui of China, while another is reminiscent of the Chinese arrangement of the five elements. The mandala was used as a teaching aid to show the various potential forces for good which exist within each of us; and also to explain the steps, to be taken to realise or manifest that inner goodness, which are experienced as a spiritual journey.

The Ziggurat

The ziggurat was a man-made sacred mountain which was used in the religion of Light/Life of early Mesopotamia and Persia. Its four corners represent the four directions of east, west, north and south. Some had seven levels, others had five or three, symbolising the steps to heaven. At the summit of the ziggurat was a palace where the chief god resided. There was another palace at the base of the ziggurat. These two palaces seem to have represented the idea of "as above, so below" and therefore the directions of above and below.

Above	=	Heaven (Positive) or (Father)
3 Steps	=	Trinity (Man in Balance) (Neutral)
5 Steps and		
7 Steps	=	Steps of a Spiritual Journey
Below	=	Earth (Negative) or (Mother)

The Ba Gua

It appears that when Buddhism moved into China it took the diagrammatical arrangements of the Five Elements and the Ba Gua familiar to the Chinese and used them as teaching aids to explain the Buddhist theories, which I find simpler and easier to understand than the equivalent Hindu arrangement of a world tree.

BA GUA   **BUDDHA LAND**

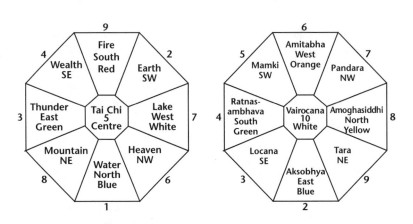

Chinese Buddhists appear to have renamed the Ba Gua "Buddha-Land" and used it to represent the journey to Buddhahood or Enlightenment. It can be applied to any kind of journey—the journey of life, a spiritual journey, learning a new skill or going through a relationship. In Taoism the journey is thought to be a kind of zig-zag pathway while in Buddhism it is seen as a circle or spiral which culminates in the centre. The Ba Gua is always shown with the direction of South at the top because it was believed that the Emperor of China always sat facing South so any map or plan placed in front of him had south at the top. When the Buddha meditated under the Bodhi tree he faced East so that direction is always in front of the Buddha seated at the centre of a mandala—therefore east is shown at the bottom of a Buddha-land. It appears to me that the Buddhists retained quite a few aspects of the Ba Gua and so a way of understanding the mandala is to envisage an invisible Ba Gua lying beneath the Buddha-Land. For example, this means that some of the qualities of the South section of the Ba Gua will be found in the West section of a Buddha land—the colours red/orange, the element Fire, and so on—and as the South section of the Ba Gua was considered the most auspicious this may be one reason why Buddha Amitabha (Buddha of the West) is so popular in Asia.

There are eight sections in a Buddha Land and each section is looked after by one of the eight Bodhisattvas, or Buddhas who assist the Buddha sitting at the centre of the Buddha Land. A land is entered in the east (Birth) and each section is travelled in a clock-wise direction (sunrise to sunset) to the eighth section in the north east. South which represents the positive polarity and summer, is shown at the top of the Ba Gua because it also represents mid-day. North, representing the negative polarity and winter, is shown at the bottom of the Ba Gua because it also represents mid-night. In Buddhism South and North appear on the horizontal axis of the mandala indicating balance of the positive/negative polarities. The mandala can represent a journey of a day, a month, a year or seven years (the east section of birth is not counted as it is considered passive).

The Old Testament of the Bible says that God made the world in six days and rested on the seventh. For Buddhists the first day of birth is a rest or passive day and the following seven are active days. Buddha Sakyamuni is said to have taken seven steps after he was born. On the third level of the Healing Buddha mandala the Great Mother represents birth, passiveness and rest, while Sakyamuni and the six Healing Buddhas represent the seven active steps of the mandala.

When students of the mandala integrate all its aspects they become "one" with the Buddha in the centre who represents the condition which the students (Bodhisattva) wish to attain or to which they want to become "enlightened". From that integration comes the "seed" or idea for a new journey and greater enlightenment. Therefore the central Buddha also acts as the "Father" of the next journey. If the students do not integrate their experiences they will travel the same journey again and again, repeating the same patterns in their life until they understand the lessons they are being presented with and how to overcome them by rejoicing in their positive achievements and letting go of their negative qualities so that they do not arise in their lives.

Some of this information is to be found in the 51-fold Healing Buddha mandala. Much of the information would have been passed on orally to the monks and this information may now be lost or may never become available to Westerners. Some of the information (as commentaries to the sutras) has yet to be translated into English or other European languages.

A "Buddha-World" is ten Buddha-Lands.

Buddha-World (The Buddha Lands of the 10 Directions)

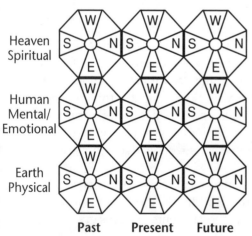

This diagram (left) only shows 8 directions—the other two directions are Above and Below—meaning that the mandalas not only align side by side but also stack one on top of the other.

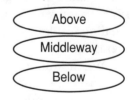

Above

Middleway

Below

Between each Buddha-Land there is a gate. At this gate there is a doorman and a guardian. They will either allow you to pass through that gate or prevent you from entering the gate. Also at each gate there is a two way mirror which enables you to see the qualities in the people you meet that are a reflection of your own life and qualities.

Fifty Buddha-Worlds equal a Buddha-Star System and a "Universe" is one hundred Buddha-Worlds which is 10 worlds x 10 directions which means that each universe contains 1,000 Central Buddhas. There are three universes—past, present and future—which make a total of 3,000 Buddhas.

The Five Elements

The Chinese arrangement of the five elements—wood, fire, earth, metal and water—uses the four quarters and the centre. The arrangement also represents the cosmos with the centre as the point towards which all intergration moves and from which the many things of the our world manifest into form.

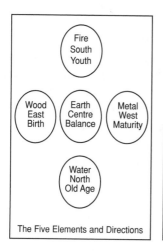

The Five Elements and Directions

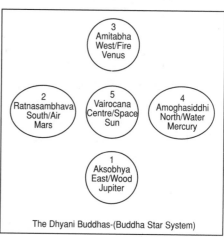

The Dhyani Buddhas-(Buddha Star System)

This "five elements" arrangement seems to represent the influence of elements, direction, planets and colour which are believed to have an effect on our lives and are personified by the Five Dhyani Buddhas—Aksobhya, Ratnasambhava, Amitabha, Amoghasiddhi and Vairocana.

This Star system arrangement represents your place in the world/universe and your relationship to others in the world/universe. It will also represent how far or close you are to your central goal.

NUMBERS

For many centuries numbers have had a metaphysical meaning because it was believed that they are the basis of, and are responsible for, the harmony of the universe. It was the appearance of numbers within the Reiki Story which made me wonder about the metaphysical aspects of the story. The metaphysical level of Reiki was later confirmed by finding symbols which can be read as "A Torch in Daylight" within the Reiki Master symbol.

Three

Three is the trinity of Heaven, Earth and Human. Heaven = positive (yang), Earth = negative (yin), Human = neutral (yin/yang). Three is the ideal. It is indivisible by an even number therefore it has no polarity. The Universal Life Force (Reiki) which brings the energy of earth and heaven together in humans has no polarity ie: Universal = Heaven; Force = Earth; Life = Human. In Reiki we say the name of a symbol, intent or affirmation three times so that it is integrated as a balanced trinity.

Seven

In most societies the number seven is considered sacred. It represents the seven steps we take from birth to

2. Symbols of Buddhism

death or from earth to heaven, which have also been described as the seven ages of humanity. The final step before death is the seventh—the time of reflection, of looking at the positive and negatives experienced during the other stages of life, of comparing your experiences with your overall principles and then either deleting, modifying or originating your principles. You may have a need to do this work in a quiet space—a monastery, a retreat, the shed at the back of the garden, your own study or den, or a sanctuary. This experience can be supported and confirmed by sacred ritual or initiation.

The number seven turns up several times within the Reiki Story. Mikao Usui was said to have studied at Chicago University for seven years. He was also said to have practiced Reiki in the Beggar City for seven years. The number seven can be used to imply the stages an initiate passes through to reach a spiritual goal. The statement that Mikao Usui did something for seven years would indicate that he went through all the stages of that experience and reached a particular spiritual goal. Which would also indicate that his experience in the Beggar City and his supposed time at Chicago University had positive results which benefited his spiritual goal. That, although he did not learn to heal with his hands at Chicago University nor did he effect a healing in the young men in the Beggar City, these experiences were viewed as positive, and by being treated as positive they benefited his spiritual goal. It is also a lesson to readers/listeners of the Reiki Story that each of us look at our failures for the positive aspects which can lead us to the next stage of our spiritual journey. The number seven can also represent the seven consciousnesses of the male aspect of God.

Eight

In Buddhism, the number eight represents the complete circle/wheel, the journey from birth to death. It represents the seven active and one passive step of the journey that leads to enlightenment. In Asia eight is a lucky number.

Ten

The Buddha at the centre of a mandala is both one and zero. The number one represents the start of your journey of a mandala—the Buddha you want to attain oneness with; the zero symbolises the complete journey—when you have achieved enlightenment or attainment or oneness with the energetic force of the Buddha. This concept in the west is found in the following quote attributed to God: "I am the alpha and the omega—the beginning and the end"

Seventeen

I believe seventeen is the vibrational number of the Universal Life Force energy we call Reiki. There are 17 spokes in the wheel which appears on the foot of the Healing Buddha at Yakushi-ji, Nara, Japan. The Japanese version of the Reiki Master symbol contains seventeen strokes; and its name is also the name of the 34th Past Buddha (17x2=34); and the mandala for the Healing Buddha is known as the 51-fold Healing Buddha Mandala (17x3=51).

THE JOURNEY

For many centuries mankind has looked upon life as a journey. When symbols and archetypes are used the journey becomes a heroic or spiritual journey in search of the soul, God-self or Buddhahood. The spiritual journey is the basic outline of most fairy stories, folk tales, myths and legends. Once a person commences that journey, either willingly or unwittingly, they are given one or more gifts to assist them in times of stress and danger.

Symbolically the journey is commenced in the East with the rising sun. The most positive point of the journey, when anything seems possible, is mid-day or mid-summer when the sun is at its zenith. Taking on the difficulty or challenge of claiming the prize or princess is seen as the west when the sun is setting. The most dangerous part of the journey is at mid-night or mid-winter when the sun is at its lowest point. The successful completion of the journey is when the Prince is united with the Princess with the approval of the King and Queen. The Prince represents Reason and Logic. The Princess represents Intuition. The King represents the positive while the Queen represents the negative. Understanding and over-coming the lessons of the journey enables the traveller to be fully balanced between negative and positive, reason and intuition, which then allows them to realise their God-self or reach Buddhahood.

The roots of Reiki appear to be connected with just such a journey. Within the Reiki system we are given gifts. The ability to connect with and channel the energy we know as Reiki, the Five Reiki Principles and four symbols. Reiki, a journey to wholistic well being, can be expressed as a Buddhist mandala which is a picture of a spiritual journey. The Buddhists recognised that there are many ways of trav-elling a spiritual journey and so developed a variety of man-dalas. The Healing Buddha's mandala is the one which has the most relevance to Reiki.

37 Natures of Enlightenment Mandala

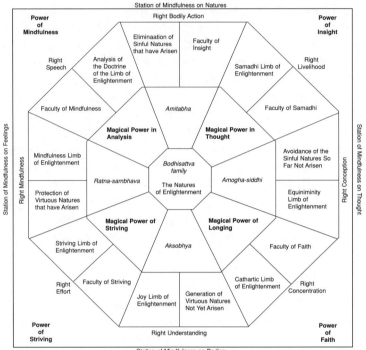

Chapter 3

The Healing Buddha Pantheon

Many years ago during a prosperity class held by a Unity minister we were told to meditate on our life path or divine plan. In one of the clearest visualisations I have ever experienced I saw a large brick wall. I tried to go around it. I tried to go over it. I could do neither so I began to dismantle the wall, one brick at a time. Behind the wall was a huge golden Buddha; the most beautiful statue I had ever seen, glowing gold and decorated with precious jewels. Although a statue, it had an energy which made it seem almost alive. The minister suggested that I read some books on Buddhism. I didn't. I did go to the library and I did select a thick, heavy book on Buddhism, but was dismayed at the weight and size of the book so I put it back on the shelf.

Several years later I heard about Reiki and just "knew" it was right for me. One thing led to another and eventually I began looking for Reiki within Buddhism so that as a Reiki Master I would have a deeper and clearer understanding of this wonderful energy we call Reiki. The process has been a bit like taking down a brick wall, brick by brick. And yes, I did find a Buddha, one who emanates divine healing rays.

The Reiki Story tells us that Reiki was rediscovered in the Buddhist records. I am convinced that Mikao Usui studied the sutras of the Healing Buddha because a description of the Reiki Master symbol can be found within the first two vows made by the Healing Buddha.

The Healing Buddha sutras, which appear in the book *The Healing Buddha* by Raoul Birnbaum, are written in such a way that at first reading they appear to be a collection of promises made by mythical/magical personalities with little relevance to Reiki or any kind of transference of a healing energy.

Buddhist sutras are written to be read (or listened to) in at least two, if not three ways. The first way was meant for lay people and the second way for the initiated—those people who become monks dedicating their lives to Buddha. The third way was for the monks who had studied the sutras for many years and could understand their hidden metaphysical messages. This metaphysical level is pursued in Japan by the Shingon and Tendai sects of Buddhism which has led some people to believe that Mikao Usui had belonged to one or the other. Although at first reading the sutras of the Healing Buddha appear to have little relevance for Reiki practitioners, after gaining some understanding of Buddhist language and its double or hidden meanings the sutras begin to take on a more vital and interesting relevance to Reiki.

The Healing Buddha's pantheon consists of a number of deities.

Main Deities	Associated Deities
The Healing Buddha	The 53 Past Buddhas
The Seven Healing Buddha Brothers	Dainichi (Vairocana)
The Bodhisattvas of Sunlight and Moonlight	The Great Mother
The Twelve Yaksha Generals	The Bodhisattva Families
	Buddhas of the 10 Directions
	Guardians of the 10 Directions
	Kings of the Four Directions

The Healing Buddha

English	=	Master of Healing, the Lapis Lazuli Radiance Tathagata
Sanskrit	=	Bhaishajyaguru Vaidurya Prabhasa Tathagata
Japanese	=	Yakushi Rurikwo Nyorai

3. The Healing Buddha Pantheon

The Healing Buddha, first recorded in Buddhist scripture around 150 AD may, according to Alexander Soper, represent Christ; having been brought to Northern India by early Christians fleeing the persecution of the Romans. This idea seems to be supported by the fact that the Healing Buddha has twelve assistants known as the 12 Yaksha Generals who, when depicted as statues, have red curly hair—a sign of their foreign (non-Asian) origins—and may represent Christ's 12 disciples. My thought is that Christ and his disciples, and the Healing Buddha and his 12 Generals, are "opposite sides of the same coin"; that Christianity is the result of the beliefs of Mesopotamia going west and Buddhism is the result of those same beliefs going east.

The Healing Buddha represents both the beginning and the end of the spiritual journey of healing. He is the "alpha and the omega"—the one and the zero. He is seated in the centre of the mandala representing complete integration with the healing energy of the universe at the cosmic level. The traditional colour of the Healing Buddha is deep blue which is said to represent unchanging reality. This deep blue is also the colour of lapis lazuli and he is also known as Master of Healing, Lapis Lazuli Radiance. From ancient times comes the belief that gemstones give off potent healing energies for which lapis lazuli was greatly valued. The Healing Buddha's name of Lapis Lazuli Radiance seems to indicate that he radiated an energy the same or similar to lapis lazuli. *(I have found that lapis lazuli (placed at any chakra point) complements Reiki well when used in a Reiki Treatment).*

The Healing Buddha, as either a statue or painting, is often seen holding a lapis lazuli medicine bowl in his left hand and a twig of the myrobalan tree in his right hand. The fruit of the myrobalan tree is said to heal the eyes; cure wounds, skin troubles, and the painful passage of urine; help digest food; make the mind attentive; and grant long life. In Buddhism the myrobalan has been used as a symbol for the creative power of thought and is said to represent blessings from unseen realms which were described as healing energy radiating on worshippers.

At other times the Healing Buddha can be seen with his hands held in "mudra" positions: the left hand, palm outwards, fingers pointing to the ground, signifying the bestowal of blessings; and the right hand, palm outwards, fingers pointing to the sky with thumb and middle finger bent slightly towards each other, signifying the banishment of fear or the bestowing of courage.

Some early Chinese descriptions of the Healing Buddha refer to him as the Healing Tree Buddha which appears to correlate his position as a Buddha of the East with the Chinese element of Tree or Wood which is found in the eastern section of a Chinese Ba Gua.

The Healing Buddha represents the healing energy of the universe, the healing energy within ourselves and the healing energy of earth all integrated and in balance with one another. Sitting at the centre of the mandala demonstrates that this energy can be brought together in unity. Reiki is the name Mikao Usui gave for this unity which is known as the Universal (Heaven) Life (Human) Force (Earth) Energy.

The Healing Buddha made twelve vows; the first two describe his subtle, energetic body and the other ten represent the various ways a person will be healed when they accept his teachings and become "one" with him. In *The Sutra of the Lord of Healing* by the Society of Chinese Buddhists, a translation of the Hsuan-tsang version (AD 650) of the Healing Buddha sutra, each of his vows begin with "*I vow that after I have been born into the world and have attained Perfect Enlightenment...*". It is my opinion that

26

3. The Healing Buddha Pantheon

"being born into the world" indicates being initiated with the Healing Buddha energy (ie: the Reiki Master symbol) and "attained Perfect Enlightenment" means the integration and flowering and expression of the stream of knowledge and energy which was passed on during the initiation.

The Seven Healing Buddhas

These Buddhas are often referred to as brothers because they are all aspects of the Healing Buddha. They appear to me to represent the Western idea that there are seven consciousnesses of God. These Healing Buddhas are often depicted as a large Healing Buddha surrounded by six small Healing Buddhas—three on the left side and three on the right side of the Healing Buddha. In Tibet and China these Healing Buddhas are also known as the Medicine Buddhas. Each Buddha is considered to be a teacher who will instruct the initiate in how to be healed. Although each Buddha teaches exactly the same lesson to each initiate because each initiate has different problems/illnesses they will experience the lessons differently. Another aspect of these Healing Buddhas is that they are all parts of the pure essence of a person. It is this essence which can become a Buddha, Tathagata or "Perfectly Enlightened One". These Buddhas are found on the third level of the Healing Buddha mandala. They are:

SE   Sakyamuni (Founder of Buddhism)

> The Buddha Sakyamuni represents the philosophy, principles and beliefs which assist the initiate through the mandala. It was said Sakyamuni could become a king or a Buddha. In the Healing Buddha mandala he appears as a king and represents a component of the Healing Buddha which heals by healing your relationship between yourself and God and your spiritual beliefs.

S   **Auspicious King, Tathagata, Arhat, Perfectly Enlightened One, Perfect in Mind and Deed, Well-gone, Tamer of Passions, He who Knows the world. (Suparikirtita-namasri)**

His body is coloured yellow; (the colour of the south section of the mandala) his right hand is held in the mudra for Teaching the Law, his left hand is held in the dhyana mudra which is the meditation gesture. His eight vows are subtle expressions of his Buddhahood. His Pure Land is known as "Radiant Victory".

SW   **Sovereign King, Majestic Light and Sound of the Moon Jewel Insight, Tathagata, Arhat, Perfectly Enlightened One. (Svaraghosa-raja)**

He has a red-yellow body and his right hand makes the gesture for Teaching the Law, and his left hand is held in the meditation mudra. He also has eight vows. It is recommended that this Buddha is worshipped and his name spoken six times during the day and night and eventually whatever is desired will become manifest. His Pure Land is known as "Marvellous Gem". (Although the Buddha situated in South direction of the mandala has the same colour as the section of the mandala where he sits, this Buddha and the following Buddhas do not. Why these Healing Buddhas are yellow, red, or red-yellow is not clear).

W   **Radiant Gem of Golden Hue, Perfected in the Sublime Practices, Tathagata, Arhat, Perfectly Enlightened One. (Suvarna-bhadra-vimala-ratna-prabhasa)**

His body is coloured red-yellow with his right hand making the Teaching the Law mudra, and his left hand held in the meditation mudra. His Pure Land is known as "Wholly Complete Incense Heap". He has four vows. He also has a dharani, which is a spiritual formula, that should be recited six times a day which will eliminate karmic fetters.

NW   **Without Grief, He Who is most Excellent and Auspicious, Tathagata, Arhat, Perfectly Enlightened One. (Asokottamasri)**

His body is light red and both hands are in the meditation mudra. His Pure Land is known as "Without Grief". He made four subtle and great vows. His name and vows should be repeated with reverence and utmost sincerity six times each day and night.

N **Thundering Sound of the Dharma Sea, Tathagata, Arhat, Perfectly Enlightened One. (Dharmakirti-sagaraghosa)**

He has a red body and holds his right hand in the bestowing blessings gesture and his left hand in the meditation gesture. His Pure Land is known as "Dharma Banner". He also has four vows. Reciting this Buddha's vows and name will ensure a long life free of illness and the necessities of life will be supplied whenever you think of them.

NE **The Buddha, Victorious Wisdom of the Dharma Sea, He who Roams Freely by His Spiritual Powers, Tathagata, Arhat, Perfectly Enlightened One. (Abhijna-raja)**

His body is red. His right hand makes the bestowal of blessings mudra and his left hand is held in the meditation gesture. His Pure Land is known as "Wholesome Abode in the Sea of Jewels". He also has four vows.

The Pure Lands of the Buddhas

Every Buddha has a "Pure Land". The Pure Lands of each of the Seven Healing Buddhas are described in the book *Healing Buddha* by Raoul Birnbaum. At the beginning of each description of a Healing Buddha the Buddha Sakyamuni states that their Pure Land is found in the East and gives a distance (related as a number of Buddha-fields) to indicate its position on the mandala. Each of the eight segments (or mountains) of the mandala is a "Pure Land". Each "Pure Land" has 4 levels—physical (Earth), mental/emotional (Human), spiritual (Heaven) and nirvana (Cosmic). Each land is peopled with a Buddha, Bodhisattvas, Guardians of Direction, and Yaksha Generals.

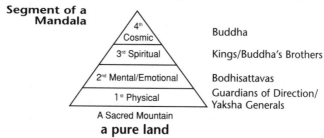

Segment of a Mandala

4th Cosmic — Buddha
3rd Spiritual — Kings/Buddha's Brothers
2nd Mental/Emotional — Bodhisattavas
1st Physical — Guardians of Direction/ Yaksha Generals

A Sacred Mountain

a pure land

The Bodhisattvas and Yaksha Generals are leaders of thousands of other Bodhisattvas and Yakshas. Pabongka Rinpoche states in *Liberation in the Palm of Your Hand* that how to visualise these Pure Lands is described in *The Sutra on the Lay-out of the Pure Fields*. He describes the Pure Lands as Merit Fields—the source of all health and happiness and that our task is to plough these fields with faith and plant them with the seeds of happiness and health.

No women are allowed in the Seven Healing Buddhas' Lands. This does not mean women are barred from becoming a Master of Healing. In this context women mean negative/passive and men mean positive/active. All the Healing Buddhas' Lands are positive/active experiences. In some mandalas Buddhas can have female partners or several lands can be allocated to female deities who represent the yin side of an experience or emotion. It is said that any woman (negative/passive person) who enters the Healing Buddha Land will be transformed into a man (positive/active person). All the deities in the Healing Buddha mandala are male except for the "Great Mother" who gives birth to the journey, the Buddhas and Bodhisattvas, and acts as a witness to enlightenment.

The qualities of the Pure Lands are the qualities of the mind that the traveller must cultivate and integrate to enable him to move on to the next land. Each land is positive, indicating that the entire mind should be positive, and its soil consists of pure lapis lazuli, which means that

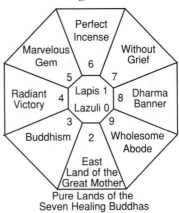

Pure Lands of the
Seven Healing Buddhas

these lands of the Seven Healing Buddhas symbolise a pure and unique aspect of the universe/mind. Being always happy, positive, non-judgmental, compassionate yet realistic is indeed unique for many people.

The Great Mother

The Goddess who appears in eastern section of the Healing Buddha mandala is a representation of the Great Mother who has many different expressions such as: The Virgin Mary, Kwan Yin, Sekhmet, Isis, Tara, Gaia, Earth Mother, Demeter, Hera, and so on. In *The Healing Buddha* the Great Mother is given the Tibetan name of "Yum-chen-mo." In *Mystic Art of Ancient Tibet* there is mention of a Medicine Goddess, known by the Sanskrit name of Bhaishajya Devi which translates to the Tibetan name of *sMan-gyi-lHa-mo*, who, in my opinion, is the feminine aspect of the Healing Buddha. The Great Mother, the only woman among the Healing Buddhas, represents the only passive area on the mandala. At the physical or first level of the mandala the Great Mother represents the conditions that cause someone to begin the journey of becoming a Master of Healing. These conditions are often negative such as illness or unhappiness; either your own or someone else's. At the other levels the Great Mother's role is to find the "arrows hidden in the heart" of an initiate. At the second level these are arrows which hurt on the mental/emotional level. At the third level they are the arrows which prevent spiritual wellness. The Great Mother also acts as a witness to your progress through the work of the mandala and may appear to the initiate during a dream or meditation where she may impart information or perform an initiation.

Although no mention is made of her in Reiki, I believe the Great Mother is a vital element of Reiki. During the process of enlightenment Buddha Sakyamuni called upon the Goddess of Earth to testify that he had accumulated only virtuous deeds in all his previous lives. When he touched the earth with the fingers of his right hand the earth opened and the Earth Goddess came to stand witness for him. I believe that one of the roles of the Great Mother within Reiki is to witness when we are ready to take the next step along the path to our enlightenment.

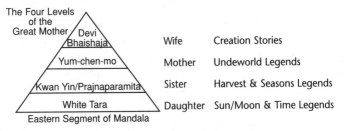

The Four Levels of the Great Mother		
Devi Bhaishaja	Wife	Creation Stories
Yum-chen-mo	Mother	Undeworld Legends
Kwan Yin/Prajnaparamita	Sister	Harvest & Seasons Legends
White Tara	Daughter	Sun/Moon & Time Legends

Eastern Segment of Mandala

For the above illustration of the Great Mother section of the Healing Buddha mandala I have chosen the White Tara for the first level because, according to David Snellgrove in *Indo-Tibetan Buddhism*, she can manifest as a Great Goddess, as a feminine version of Avalokitesvara who appears on the second level of the Healing Buddha mandala, or as his daughter. The White Tara is known to bestow long life and heal 404 diseases. There are 21 versions of Tara indicating that she belongs on the first level of a mandala.

Originally there were no female Bodhisattvas or Buddhas in Buddhism. When Buddhism arrived in China, where the philosophy of Yin and Yang (passive/active) balance had already been around for centuries, the concept of men who could be either passive or active was not readily accepted so consequently the passive Buddhas and Bodhisattvas became female. Avalokitesvara became Kwan Yin in China, Tara in Tibet and Kwannon in Japan.

3. THE HEALING BUDDHA PANTHEON

On the second level I have placed Kwan Yin, the Chinese female version of Avalokitesvara, and Prajnaparamita who as a goddess is associated with Manjushri, the other Bodhisattva to be found at this level of the mandala.

In the Healing Buddha sutras there is no mention of a Great Mother Goddess, however in the *Sutra on the Merits of the Fundamental Vows of the Seven Buddhas of Lapis Lazuli Radiance, the Masters of Healing* which can be found in *The Healing Buddha* by Raoul Birnbaum, the eighth deity mentioned is Vajradhara. Although he is referred to as a Bodhisattva, Vajradhara means King of the Thunderbolt and as a king belongs to the third level of a mandala. In paintings Vajradhara is dark blue, the colour of the eastern (feminine) section of the mandala, and is said to be so lost in divine meditation that he does not get directly involved in the affairs of sentient beings. This seems to indicate that Vajradhara is passive and therefore, like Avalokitesvara, may have a feminine version in China and Japan. In Tibet this version seems to be the Great Mother, Yum-chen-mo. In the sutra Vajradhara promises to answer questions, speak to people in dreams and cause desires to be fulfilled.

The Bodhisattva Families

A Bodhisattva is an "Enlightened Being" and is found on the second level of a mandala. Apart from Manjushri (Gentle Glory) and Avalokitesvara (Observer of the Cries of the World), each of the Bodhisattvas shown on the Healing Buddha mandala are leaders of a family. Combined, these families make up the energy of the second level of the mandala. Each family consists of 37 Beings who represent the 37 natures or components which are accessories to healing and enlightenment. The 37 natures include 4 Door Guardians, 8 Goddesses, 8 Directions, 16 Bodhisattvas and 1 leader. Each family represents a lunar month = ie 29 days (the 8 Goddesses are counted as one and are evoked during an initiation. The 1 leader represents all members of the Bodhisattva family coming together as one energy and is not counted). Being the leader of a family also indicates they are tenth level Bodhisattvas—meaning they have reached enlightenment.

At the beginning of the sutra for the Seven Healing Buddhas it says that 36,000 Bodhisattva-mahasattvas were among those who gathered around the Buddha as he expounded his teaching about the Healing Buddha. I believe that every number in the sutras is important and acts as a pointer to other information. A zero represents the completion of a journey. Within a mandala there are three journeys represented by the first three circles of the mandala, therefore 36,000 Bodhisattvas means 36 entities of a mandala which represents a Bodhisattva family. These Bodhisattva families were probably so familiar to early Buddhists that it was not necessary to give a full explanation of them in the Healing Buddha sutra, but today it is difficult to discover who and what each of the families are, and how to work with them. The "Holder of the Thunderbolt's" family, also known as the Vajra or Diamond family, is displayed as a mandala in *Indo-Tibetan Buddhism Vol I*. There is a similar mandala for the Mt Meru family in *The Buddhist Tantras*.

A mandala is always worked from the outside to the centre, so a Reiki programme using the Bodhisattvas would start with the Four Door Guardians and work inwards to the centre of the mandala. As each family is a mandala and therefore a complete energy in itself, the student is obliged to "leap" from one family (energy) to the next. That leap is made during an initiation. Bodhisattva initiations are not done by Reiki Masters in the West. Initiations to some of the Bodhisattvas are available from Tibetan Lamas who often visit Western Buddhist monasteries. Most of these Lamas work with the energies of Buddha Amitabha and will initiate people to the energies of Manjusri (Gentle Glory), Maitreya (Loving Kindness), Vajrapani (Thunderbolt-in-the-hands) and the Green Tara.

The concept of the Bodhisattva families appears to be based on the idea that our mental attitudes and emotions have a number of components which build into a unit similar to a family unit. Also like a family unit, they may not always get along with one another very well. The aim of healing on the second level of the mandala is to ensure these families of attitudes and emotions work together as one unit in harmony and to benefit the person concerned. Hence one of the Bodhisattva vows is to "ensure happiness and good fortune for all living beings".

The other thing of note with these families is that to enter them you must first pass the Doorman and then the Guardian, which can explain why getting into your attitudes and emotions can sometimes prove difficult—when you have found the password that gets you past the Doorman you are then met by the Guardian, who will not let you through until you have the right key. When you pass the Guardian you then move into the area where your thoughts/attitudes and emotions are held which, when they work for your highest good, are known as Bodhisattvas, which means Enlightened Beings.

It has been impossible to discover all the Bodhisattva families who are depicted in the Healing Buddha mandala. This information probably has to wait until someone translates into English the sastras and commentaries for the Healing Buddha sutras which are most likely to be found in ancient Buddhist monasteries in Japan.

The Bodhisattvas of Sunlight and Moonlight

English	*Sunlight*	*Moonlight*
Sanskrit	*Suryaprabha*	*Candraprabha*
Japanese	*Nikko*	*Gakko*

Also known as Solar Radiance and Lunar Radiance, the Bodhisattvas of Sunlight and Moonlight are the Guardians of the Healing Buddha's Correct Law. The Correct Laws represent the natural laws of the universe; therefore the Healing Buddha's Correct Law is the natural law of the healing energy of the universe, the immutable laws concerning the healing energy.

These two are the principle Bodhisattvas of the Healing Buddha because as Sunlight (positive) and Moonlight (negative) they, together with the Healing Buddha (neutral), form a trinity. Their Japanese characters can be found within the Reiki Master symbol. Esoterically Sunlight symbolises the Light Energy of the Universe—all the light in the universe, whether it comes from a sun, a star or a moon is sunlight or light from a sun. The light from the sun is hot and therefore seen as active and positive while moonlight is cool and therefore passive and negative.

In Buddhism Sunlight means Supreme Wisdom and Moonlight means Supreme Compassion. Both are of equal importance. Wisdom without compassion is knowledge without understanding, and compassion without wisdom is unwise conduct.

One of the major functions of these Bodhisattvas is to protect the healing energy from being used for evil. If anyone should try to send evil/negative intentions to someone by using the healing energy (Reiki) these Bodhisattvas promise they will turn the energy about so that it returns to the sender and heals them first. Once that has been done the energy will be sent to the intended person and it will heal them as well. These Bodhisattvas will then ensure that the relationship between the two people concerned is healed. This concept seems to go hand-in-hand with the idea that Reiki heals the practitioner first before it flows on to the receiver during a Reiki treatment or Distance Healing.

In the East the right hand is known as the Sun hand and the left hand is known as the Moon hand, so it can be assumed that Sunlight and Moonlight also symbolise radiance (light) coming from the right and left hands.

The Twelve Yaksha Generals

Time is one of the great healers. The cycles of the sun and moon are ways of symbolising time in our world ie: moon = month and sun = year = 12 months. The Twelve Yaksha Generals represent time. They appear in the 51-Fold Healing Buddha mandala in conjunction with the Guardians of the Ten Directions, who represent place, symbolising that time and place are in harmony.

On one occasion in the sutras it states that each General had 7,000 troops yet later it states that each General had 84,000 troops. The numbers appear to represent years and months, as well as the ten directions and one hundred Buddha-worlds. For example:

7 years x 12 months = 84 months

Add in the ten directions

7 years x 10 directions = 70 (A person's allotted
life-span) x 12 = 840 months

Add in the one hundred worlds (representing the number of journeys in a lifetime) and the result is:

(7 years x 10 directions x 100 worlds) = 7,000 x 12 = 84,000

Seventy years symbolises the length of a person's life. The 12

Yaksha Generals promise to protect people who believe in the Healing Buddha no matter where they are and ensure that they live out their allotted span of life. The number 7,000 can also be interpreted as the seven active steps of the mandala on all three levels, physical, mental/emotional, and spiritual, and therefore could mean that the promises of the Yaksha Generals pervade all three levels of the mandala.

The 12 Yaksha Generals (time) plus the 10 Directions (place) ensure you are in the right place at the right time which means that you do not meet up with an untimely death, described in the Healing Buddha sutras as being caused by:

1. Untreated illness; or wrong medicine given for an illness; or illness treated by hoodoo.

2. Execution according to the ruler's laws.

3. A person who goes out on hunts or pleasure excursions and engages in debauchry and drunkenness (ie: drunken driving).

4. Death by fire.

5. Drowning.

6. Being devoured by wild beasts.

7. Falling off a mountain precipice.

8. Harm from poisonous herbs, hateful spells, magical incantations.

9. Starvation and dehydration.

These deaths can be either literal or symbolise the various attitudes which can cause death. For example "falling off a mountain peak" represents a death brought about by loss of face, shame or loss of pride while "starvation and dehydration" represents abilities, talents and so on which go unsatisfied and unrealised. The Yaksha Generals are also known as "nature spirits" and they symbolise our innate nature, natural spirit, natural inclinations, talents and potentials.

The 12 Yaksha Generals promised to benefit and enrich all sentient beings and to bring them peace and joy no matter where they dwell. This seems to be part of what enables Reiki to be sent as absent healing no matter where a person dwells. A Kanji character for time, which the Yaksha Generals represent, can be found within Reiki's Distance symbol. They also promised that all desires would be fulfilled if a person holds to, reveres and worships the Healing Buddha. Holding the symbols of Reiki as sacred, I believe, is a way to revere the Healing Buddha.

The Ten Directions

In Buddhism the ten directions are recognised as east, south, west, north and southeast, southwest, northwest, northeast as well as above (zenith) and below (nadir). Each direction has a Buddha and a Guardian. The ten directions represent "place". Being in the "right place" at the "right time" is an important element of our health and happiness.

The Buddhas of the Ten Directions

A mandala can represent a person's life, an energy or a spiritual journey. The Buddha at the centre of that mandala symbolises the pure essence of that person, energy or journey. This effectively means that each one of us is a Buddha and our journey through life from birth to death is a mandala. The Buddhas of the Ten Directions therefore represent all those people we come into contact with each day and during our lifetimes. Each person has within them the capacity to become a Buddha. In the west this equates to recognising the God within each of us and is a way of honouring each person we meet.

The Guardians of the Ten Directions

The Guardians of the Ten Directions represent our relationships and the attitudes, inhibitions and guards we have towards relationships. These guardians each hold a mirror which reflects both the negative and positive aspects of the people we meet which can also be found within ourselves. Phases such as; "that looks like hard work", "I'm bored", "that's too hard" or "I'm not bright enough" or "no-one ever takes any notice of me" or "I've got two left feet", which are often long held excuses, can act as guardians which prevent you from pursuing a talent or opportunity or having a good relationship with friends and loved ones. When these guardians are healed they become: right understanding, right effort, right mindfulness, right speech, right bodily action, right livelihood, right concentration and right conception.

Dainichi (Vairocana)

Dainichi is the Japanese name for Vairocana (Great Sun) who is the central figure of esoteric Buddhism. This Buddha represents the Buddha within us—our central core (soul)—the creative force of the universe which can be found within each of us, often known in the west as the "Light of God Within." Dainichi is identified with enlightenment and the illuminated mind and is sometimes referred to as the "Great Illuminator". He is the idealisation of universal truth as well as being the law of the universe. All things in the universe are said to be of this Buddha. Dainichi is the point from which all form is manifested and to which all things return. Seen at the centre of the mandala, Dainichi represents the moment of integration and enlightenment. Dainichi also represents the light of the soul or pure essence of a person.

The Past Buddhas

The Past Buddhas, of which there are 53, are believed to have evolved from the twenty-four sacred names of God.

3. The Healing Buddha Pantheon

Alexander Soper states in his book *Literary Evidence for Early Buddhist Art in China* that these Buddhas cannot be explained in either time or space, but they are important and are a source of the highest power.

Because of their ability to "awaken and enlighten" the 53 Past Buddhas can impart initiatory knowledge which is essential for the progress of a spiritual journey. Another role of the Past Buddhas is to assist you to meet the right people (other Buddhas) who will help you on your spiritual journey; and you will be available at the right time and place to help others on their journey. They will assist you in remaining positive and will eliminate obstructions in your life caused by faults such as slander, disobedience and rebelliousness.

The 53 Past Buddhas are said to have held the knowledge of Buddhism for aeons of time until Sakyamuni became the Buddha. The name of the 34th Past Buddha is also the name of the Reiki Master symbol and is therefore, I believe, the holder of the knowledge of Reiki.

Guardian Kings of the Four Directions

A mandala has a gateway at each of the four directions—east, south, west and north. At each gate there is a doorman who will prevent entry if that person does not have the correct passwords. These doormen are ranked as Kings so the four directions are called realms or continents by Buddhists. Basically the doorman is the personification of the attitudes and feelings we have towards other people. Your attitude towards your parents, in particular your mother, will determine how you react to any mentors, teachers and guides in your life. If you never listened to your mother or disregarded her wisdom and advice you will treat others who share their wisdom and advice with you in the same way. Your attitude to receiving advice may also prevent you from accessing help and guidance from your Past Buddhas and Spiritual Guides. The rank of King indicates how powerful our attitudes towards other people can be.

The Five Reiki Principles act as the passwords, which open the gates of the four directions allowing harmony and a positive exchange of energy between yourself and the people you meet, either briefly or who have a long term place in your life. Once you have overcome/healed the conditions you have placed upon the Guardians of the Four Directions you can then allow these Guardians to work for you the way they are supposed to.

Direction	King	Role
East	Dhritarashtra	Purifies the thoughts and brings tranquillity
South	Virudhaka	Protects the root of goodness in humans
West	Virupaksha	Holds the power to fulfill all desires
North	Vaishravana	Protects the Buddha within

The Bodhisattva Brothers of Healing

Alexander Soper, in *Literary Evidence of Early Buddhist Art in China*, supports the idea that the Bodhisattva Brothers of Healing (King of Healing and Supreme Healer) could have derived from the Greek gods of healing, The Dioscuri, arriving in Northern India via Alexander the Great. These Bodhisattvas, also known as King of Medicine and Supreme Medicine, do not belong in the Healing Buddha mandala, even though they appear in the book *The Healing Buddha* by Raoul Birnbaum. They belong to the third level of the mandala for Amitabha, the Buddha of the Pure Land of the West also known as the Buddha of Infinite Light.

Abhiseka

A Buddhist initiation or consecration is called an Abhiseka. Very little is written about them—Raoul Birnbaum gives a only brief description in his book *The Healing Buddha*. Monks who were initiated to the energy of the Healing Buddha pledged never to reveal the secrets of the mandala and the oral teachings they had received from the Lama/Abbot. Some Tibetan Tantric initiations have appeared in print but because they have been written in the Buddhist terminology which has esoteric/hidden meanings they can be difficult to understand. Several are described in *Indo-Tibetan Buddhism Vol 1*. An Abhiseka is often represented symbolically as a waterfall or as washing the body and putting on new clothes.

The Fifty-one Fold Healing Buddha Mandala

This mandala represents all the concepts of the energy which are personified as the Healing Buddha. The 51 beings depicted in the mandala are said to be the 51 states of consciousness affiliated with healing. It was used as a teaching aid for the monks who learned about the divine healing radiance which, I believe, we now know as Reiki.

The initiates learn the mandala from the outside to the centre. The people who were initiated to the equivalent of 1st Degree Reiki learned about the Four Directions and their Guardian Kings, the Guardians of the 10 Directions, and the 12 Yaksha Generals. Those who reached 2nd Degree level would have integrated the energies of the 16 Bodhisattvas and their families and at 3rd Degree they would have learned about the inner wheel of the mandala and integrated the energies of the Seven Healing Buddhas and the Great Mother. At the 4th level the initiates would understand the message of the mandala on all levels—physical, mental/emotional, spiritual and cosmic. They would have worked through all the steps of the journey and integrated all the information of the mandala so that it became second nature to them. Much of the knowledge held within the mandala would have been passed on orally.

Outside the Mandala

Around the outside of the mandala there is a ring of flames. These flames indicate that to enter the mandala will bring about a transformation so complete that nothing of our old self remains. The mandala is then bounded by a narrow band of blue and then a band of white which contains sixteen golden thunderbolts (vajras). When placed in the outer circle of a mandala the vajras symbolise the determination and commitment needed to reach the centre of the mandala. Next comes a ring of lotus petals which symbolises the transcendental; of rising to a positive mental state and full awareness of reality. The lotus petals also signify rebirth on a higher level.

The Four Gates

The inner area of a mandala represents the house or palace of a Buddha. To enter this area you must pass through a gate. There are four gates which are aligned to the four directions of East, South, West and North. It is usual to enter a mandala at the East gate, which is found at the bottom of the mandala. At each gate there is a guardian who protects the mandala from negative energy. They will also block you from leaving the mandala, if you lose heart or become fearful, once you have entered it. Whoever they allow to enter the mandala they will protect. Above each gate sit a pair of deer. These animals sit only when it is safe, therefore they are symbols which tell us that it is safe to enter this mandala.

Outer Ring of the Mandala—The First Turning of the Wheel (Equal to 1st Degree Reiki)

Inside the four gates of the mandala is the first ring of the mandala composed of twenty-two white petals, each with blue tips, with a symbol on them. Feng Shui uses blue and white together to signify "helpful people". These symbols represent the Twelve Yaksha Generals and the Guardians of the Ten Directions; time and place. These numbers can be found in Reiki as the 12 hand positions and the ten digits of the hands. They represent the physical level of the energy encompassed within the mandala.

Second Ring of the Mandala—The Second Turning of the Wheel (Equal to 2nd Degree Reiki)

The sixteen petals of the second circle of the mandala are deep red with green tips. Feng Shui uses the colours red and green together to represent fortunate blessings. These petals can contain either the symbols or images of the sixteen Bodhisattvas. They are:

Direction	*Name*	*Symbol*	*Purpose*
East	Manjushri Gentle Glory	sword & book	Cuts thru blocks to wisdom
	Avalokitesvara Observer of the Cries of the World	lotus	Compassion
	Vajrapani Holder of the Thunderbolt	thunderbolt	Overcomes fear, cuts to reality
	Suryaprabha Sunlight	sun	Healing/wisdom
South	Candraprabha Moonlight	moon	Healing/Joy/compassion
	Mahamati Great Wisdom	eye	Wisdom from Observation
	Maitreya Loving Kindness	lotus	Good humour/good luck/karma
	Nagavrksa Clear Wisdom	book on lotus	Wisdom of Tree (pattern) of Life

Direction	Name	Symbol	Purpose
West	Pratibhanakuta Eloquent Peak	incense vessel	Right use of mind
	Rnams-par gnon-po Unfailing Transcendence	sword	Courage
	Darsaniya Well Appearing	book on lotus	Worth and Beauty
	Mun-pa thams-cad nges par Grasps the Wondrous Mountain Peak	jewel-stick	Wisdom which conquers Obscurity
North			
	Bsam-pa legs-par bsam-pa Ever Reflecting	vase of amrta	Having the right thoughts
	Merukuta Summit of Eloquence	crescent on lotus	Automatically doing things well
	Sang-sang-pa'i dbyangs Subtle and Wondrous Voice	thunderbolt	Eloquence of Language
	Merusikhara Mountain Peak	vase of amrta	Body and Mind harmony

*At the beginning of the Sutra for the Seven Healing Buddhas are listed the names, in English, of fourteen Bodhisattvas. I have applied these names, plus Sunlight and Moonlight, Chief Bodhisattvas of the Healing Buddha, to the sixteen Sanskrit/ Tibetan Bodhisattvas whose names appear in the material on the Mandala in the book *The Healing Buddha* by Raoul Birnbaum.

These sixteen Bodhisattvas represent the mental/emotional qualities which will assist both the healing and the healer. Each in turn would have been meditated on their qualities and practiced until the initiated "lived" or experienced them daily without effort. It should be noted that Mikao Usui is said to have learned several languages and also to have been courageous. It is interesting to note that both these qualities can be found within the second level of the Healing Buddha mandala.

3. The Healing Buddha Pantheon

Some of the symbols which accompany these Bodhisattvas are Buddhist versions of the Reiki symbols and it is possible that they indicate which symbols to use when you want to heal or activate a particular quality represented by a Bodhisattva. ie:

Thunderbolt	=	Power symbol	Lotus	= Mental/Emotional symbol
Book	=	Distance symbol	Vase	= Master symbol
Sun & Moon	=	Hands-on Reiki	= Sun (right hand) and Moon (left hand)	

Therefore "crescent with lotus," for instance, could mean drawing the Mental/Emotional symbol with the left hand or placing the Mental/Emotional symbol on the left hand during a Reiki treatment.

Third Ring of the Mandala—Third Turning of the Wheel (Equal to 3rd Degree Reiki)

In this circle are Six Healing Buddhas, Sakyamuni and the Great Mother who teach how to integrate the passive and active aspects of the energetic force of the Healing Buddha. They sit in eight petals coloured light red with white tips which in Feng Shui represent intimate relationships or marriage. This level marries together the 1st level and the 2nd level and integrates the energies of those levels into one energy.

The Centre of the Mandala—Nirvana (would be equal to 4th Degree of Reiki)

At the centre of the mandala sits the Master of Healing. At this level, the cosmic level, the initiate achieves "oneness" with the Master of Healing and completely integrates the healing energy. The initiate is now completely healed and remains in balance regardless of what experience or person comes into their life. Mikao Usui's experience at the top of the mountain and Sakyamuni's experience under the bodhi tree indicate that this integration with the energy held at the centre of the mandala is an actual physical experience which happens when all the work of the mandala has been done.

HEALING BUDDHA MANDALA

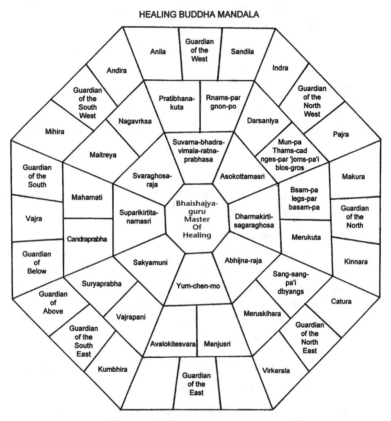

The Symbols on the Hand and Foot of the Healing Buddha

(photos of the hand and foot appear in *"Japanese Temples"* by J Edward Kidder Jr)

On a hand and foot of the statue of the Healing Buddha

at Yakushi-ji, Nara, Japan are etched symbols. The etchings tell the story of a spiritual journey. On the foot the message is read from the heel to the toes. The symbol in the hand denotes the culmination of the journey which is integration, enlightenment, and expression of the knowledge gained.

Symbols on the Foot

The four flames which surround the small wheel on the heel represents the four gates and their doormen who must be passed before entry into the journey, and indicating it is a transformative journey.

The small wheel has ten spokes and represents the Guardians and Buddhas of the Ten Directions; all those people and conditions you will meet, influence, or be influenced by, during your journey

The trisula (the three bunches of leaves) represent the trinity of Heaven, Man and Earth being held in balance and unity. This is a major aim of the journey as well as being a major tool to assist the traveller to stay on their pathway. In Buddhism this trinity is also referred to as The Three Precious Jewels—the Buddha, the Sangha (community) and the Dharma (the teachings).

The large wheel in the centre of the foot represents the Healing Buddha mandala, which is denoted by the circle of fire and the seventeen spokes. The fire represents the transformation that can be brought about by the energy encompassed within the mandala.

The four symbols on the pad of the foot represent the tools of the journey. The conch shell under the little toe symbolises the sound of God. The vase under the next toe represents the knowledge and fruitfulness of life. The pair of fish indicate the union of yin/yang and the ability to go anywhere without constraint or restriction. The vajra under the big toe represents the diamond world of reality. The placement of these four symbols indicates whether they are yin or yang. The vajra is on the right side of the foot and is therefore yang, the conch shell is on the left side of the foot indicating it is yin. Being in the middle indicates that the fish and vase have no duality, denoting a balance of yin/yang.

All the Reiki symbols are represented on the foot:

The Vase	=	Reiki Master symbol
Vajra	=	Power symbol
Conch shell	=	Mental/Emotional symbol
Pair of fish	=	Distance symbol

The swastikas on the toes are the steps of the journey around the four directions. The flame on the big toe signifies enlightenment and transformation gained from experiences of the journey.

Symbol on the Hand

The wheel on the hand of the Healing Buddha has nine sections which represents Buddhahood; the whole journey. The pairs of strokes in the wheel symbolise positive and negative with the small circles in the wheel indicating that they are being held in unity and therefore balance. Around the outside of the wheel are twelve lotus, telling us that it is now time for the experience and knowledge gained during the journey of the mandala to be expressed in daily life.

Chapter 4

THE TWELVE HAND POSITIONS

The twelve hand positions are taught during 1st Degree Reiki classes. Because the understanding of why there are twelve hand positions has been either lost down through the lineages, or was never originally taught by Mrs. Takata, there have been many additions to the number of hand positions—some Reiki Masters teach up to twenty seven hand positions or more. Mikao Usui didn't use or teach the twelve hand positions. It is believed that Chujiro Hayashi added them to the Reiki system, which means they could have come from another healing system used in Japan during the 1920s.

As already mentioned, the number twelve relates to time and the 12 Yaksha Generals. Originally it was taught that each hand position was held for five minutes. The number five is associated with the five meditation Buddhas who represent the journey to Buddhahood. The three parts of the body—head, front, and back—form a trinity signifying the need for the body to be in balance. I believe the head represents the future, the front of the body represents the present and the back represents the past.

Our right hand symbolises yang energy which is also known as active, positive or sun energy and our left hand symbolises yin energy known as passive, negative or moon energy. Placing our hands so that they are lying across the body, one in front of the other, indicates that balance of yin/yang is required during a Reiki Treatment.

There are four hand positions on the head, another four on the front of the body and four on the back of the body. The number four represents the four parts of the Life Force Energy. These are represented in Buddhism as the four gateways and the Buddhas of the four directions—east, south, west and north. The four components of the Life Force Energy are: peace; wisdom or knowledge; compassionate love or unconditional love; and insight or psychic energy. The four hand positions symbolise bringing all the components of the Universal Life Force Energy into the treatment on all three levels.

Buddhists apply the Ten Directions, which on one level also means "place" and on another represents relationships, to the ten digits of our hands. The twelve hand positions, symbolising the Twelve Yaksha Generals, represent time and also our animal nature and untamed attitudes. A Reiki treatment will bring time and place, and relationships and attitudes, into harmony which means we find ourselves being in the "right place at the right time" therefore bringing an improvement to our relationships and our attitudes. It will also help us to confront and alter our relationships with others making us aware of our attitudes and enabling us to change our attitudes.

Pabongka Rinpoche in *Liberation in the Palm of Your Hand* describes two hand positions, similar to Reiki hand positions, and their meanings—hands on the throat to achieve enlightened speech and on the heart to gain an enlightened mind—indicating that the Healing Buddha monks probably had more "spiritual" reasons for the hand positions than just healing chakras or the endocrine system. He also says that keeping your hands flat and fingers together (which is recommended when giving a Reiki treatment), helps to achieve "webs of light between the fingers"—one of the marks of a Buddha.

4. THE TWELVE HAND POSITIONS

The Cycle of Energy

Eastern philosophy records that the Life Force Energy, known in Japan as Ki and in China as Ch'i, goes through cycles. One of the cycles used to explain the flow of the Life Force Energy is the cycle of seasons.

Regular Reiki treatments will bring you into alignment with the seasons. It seems that being in tune with the seasons is important for health and wellbeing. If you study ancient religions, this cycle of the seasons was considered important and was also held to be sacred. Being in 'tune' with the seasons means the Life Force Energy is able to flow easily into all aspects of your life and your progress along life's path becomes more natural and easier.

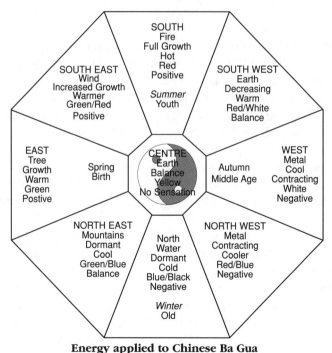

Energy applied to Chinese Ba Gua

Sensations in the Hands

The different sensations that Reiki Practitioners can experience in their hands during a Reiki treatment can be explained by the Ba Gua above. If the hands are hot when giving Reiki then the body receiving the energy is out of balance by being too yang, the problem has been there a short time and is related to the person's growth and progress. If the hands are cold then that area of the body's energy is out of balance by being too yin, the problem has been around for a long time and is related to something deep within (or dormant within) the person.

Re-educating the Body Cells

Every cell in our body is a living being. A cell is a microcosm of the whole body and contains its own memory, intelligence and function. A cell can retain the memory of any hurt or trauma it has experienced and will utilise this memory when responding to any further real or imagined hurt or trauma. This response can manifest in the body as an allergy or as pain or depression. If a hurt or trauma is dramatic enough or regular enough the cells in the body will respond automatically, like Pavlov's dogs when they heard a bell ring. For instance, when someone gets angry they may also feel a pain in their chest area, or if they are worried their body may respond with a squeezing, twisting feeling in their lower abdomen.

From my experience I believe that one of the aspects of 1st Degree Reiki is re-educating the body and all the cells in the body. This is done by channelling Reiki to various parts of the body. This re-education can also be assisted by chanting the Five Reiki Principles to yourself, over and over again at each hand position and by starting each Reiki Treatment with an intent (a statement indicating what you want healed).

Becoming OM

During a Reiki treatment the receiver often begins snoring, and their reaction is to try to stop, especially if one of the people giving the treatment makes a comment or snickers about the snoring.

When people receive Reiki they often enter into three kinds of consciousness at the same time. First their body goes to sleep, causing their breathing to change, which often results in snoring or other sounds as they begin breathing through their mouth. At the same time their minds are wide awake and they are aware they are snoring, they can hear themselves. They can also hear everything else in the room as well. Often their hearing becomes very acute, but because their bodies are asleep, and therefore their throats are asleep, they have little or no wish to respond to what is being said during the treatment. Their attention is more than likely focused on what is happening in their mind's eye (third eye) where they often see colours or images, very much like observing a dream.

This state of consciousness where the body is asleep, the mind is awake and yet they are dreaming is the ideal for a Reiki treatment. This state of consciousness is described in the symbol for the sacred sound of OM.

The first semi-circle on the OM symbol represents being awake and it is connected to the second semi-circle of sleep. Across a small gap is the semi-circle which represents the state

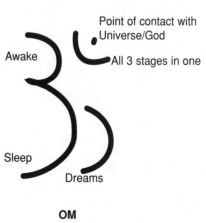

Point of contact with Universe/God

All 3 stages in one

Awake

Sleep

Dreams

OM

of dreaming. The gap symbolises that moment, just as you are dropping off to sleep, when you feel you have stepped off into nothing and your foot jerks, waking you suddenly with a fright and is perhaps why, in old children's stories, going to the "Land of Dreams" was often depicted as sailing across space towards some distant star. Dreams are important for our "Self" discovery. They process and integrate information that we have gathered during our waking periods by erasing or reinforcing information needed for our survival. In Buddhism it is said that dreaming is an active means of attaining enlightenment and is complementary to the work done while awake to attain enlightenment. Dreams are said to originate from the total human which resides in 'radiant light'. Going into a light dream state during a Reiki treatment helps us to integrate the energy more effectively and allows the energy to reach right to our essence or total self.

The semi-circle at the top of the symbol denotes that all three states, awake, sleep and dreaming have become one state, ie: the person is doing them all together at the same time, as can happen in a Reiki treatment. Both Hindus and Buddhists believe that when you enter into this state of consciousness you are able to connect with the power of the universe. The sound of OM is said to represent the sound of the universe. The small dot in the symbol represents that moment of connection with the unexplainable power of the universe to which we often give the name of God.

The Levels

Reiki practitioners are taught that Reiki heals on all levels. These levels are most often referred to as the physical, mental, emotional and spiritual. It would appear that the mental/emotional is one level and having a Reiki symbol which encompasses both of these levels as one

(Mental/Emotional Symbol) supports this idea. The fourth level is, I believe, the cosmic level. It is the level referred to in Buddhism as Nirvana, Void or Emptiness. Although it has no symbols and no form it can be experienced. In Reiki this level is experienced when either the receiver or Reiki practitioner feels they are drifting into a deep silence and have no wish to talk; their hands feel as though they have melted into the body of the receiver, with no barrier between them; and there is no conscious awareness of time passing, it is as though they have stepped outside of time. This is an ideal state to be in when either giving or receiving Reiki. It is that point of contact with the universe, of going beyond OM.

The Physical Level is our relationship with the outer physical world; people, things, the environment, animals and our body. Buddhists refer to this level as Body.

The Mental/Emotional Level is our relationship with our inner world of thoughts, attitudes, beliefs and emotions. It also incorporates the expression of our inner world. The Buddhists refer to this level as Mind.

The Spiritual Level is our explanation/thoughts about aspects of our life which cannot be experienced by our five senses but can be experienced with our mind such as the laws of nature, God, telepathy, coincidence, apparitions, auras, channelling, etc. Buddhists refer to this level as Spirit. This level is a non-dualistic combination of Body and Mind.

The Cosmic Level is the unexplainable which is the origin of all that is known and explainable—that from which we come and to which we return. Buddhists refer to this level as Void, Emptiness or Nirvana.

The three degrees of Reiki are based on the trinity of physical, mental/emotional, and spiritual. When each of these degrees are integrated the Reiki practitioner should experience the cosmic level of Reiki.

The idea of each level is to work through all aspects of the degree together so that they become one activity ie: (channel energy, use hand positions and think/say 5 Reiki Principles at the same time) so that eventually all levels of the physical degree of Reiki are integrated as one.

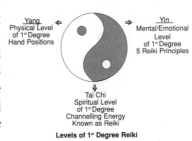

Levels of 1ˢᵗ Degree Reiki

This would indicate that the three symbols of 2nd Degree can also be used together to create an integrated and balanced mental and emotional level.

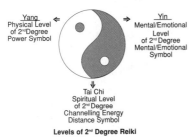

Levels of 2ⁿᵈ Degree Reiki

Each Reiki symbol should be worked with and used until the Reiki practitioner feels as though they have become 'one' with the symbol—so that there is no feeling of separateness from the symbol.

Because the spiritual level is about integrating both the physical and mental/emotional levels so they are in balance and harmony with each other there is only one symbol at Master level. This symbol integrates the yang and yin levels of spirituality so they become Tai Chi (Great Energy) or one energy.

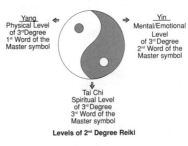

Levels of 2ⁿᵈ Degree Reiki

58

Chapter 5

THE FIVE BUDDHAS

Just for Today, Do Not Anger
Just for Today, Do Not Worry
Honour Your Parents, Teachers and Elders
Earn Your Living Honestly
Show Gratitude to all Living Beings

Mikao Usui

Early Japanese Emperors had a set of codes by which they ruled called the Ritsuryo (penal and civil) codes which were based on the Confucian principle of benevolent rule. Provincial officials toured their areas of jurisdiction to teach (among other things) the population to follow the five basic moral precepts set forth in Confucian doctrine. In 1867 it was decided that Japan would no longer be ruled by a shogun, and power was handed to Emperor Meiji who restored the imperial rule and direct rule of emperor by constitutional government in 1868. Probably following the example of his earlier ancestors, he issued five principles or precepts, which seem to have a strong Buddhist influence, for the people of Japan to live by. Apparently it is these five principles that Mikao Usui added into the Reiki system and which have become known in the west as the Five Reiki Principles.

The Reiki principles have been interpreted in a number of ways by other Reiki Masters. The best way to get a clear understanding of these principles is to work with them yourself, taking notice of how you respond to them.

It is my opinion that these principles act as passwords to remove the inhibitions, blind spots, and negative attitudes which prevent us from experiencing the best in our various types of relationships with other people. It seems to me that the first two principles work on the physical level (our outward response), the third and fourth principles work on the mental/emotional level (our inner response) and the fifth principle works on the spiritual level (the combination of both our inner and outward worlds).

It should be noted that the first two principles have no personal pronoun in them. The messages of these two principles are not directed at anyone in particular. Therefore, I believe they are designed to reach both the ego and the soul or spirit at the same time. This starts the process of the ego and soul acting together as one unit. The third and fourth principles contain the pronoun "your" signifying that these principles are directed at someone, who I believe is the ego/soul unit which by joining together have become another entity other than themselves. The fifth principle also has no pronoun, indicating to me that it is designed to reach both the ego/soul unit and beyond the ego/soul unit to the part of our being which is also part of the cosmos.

It is said there are three obstacles which prevent you from travelling a spiritual path. They are hate, fear and indecision. The five Reiki Principles are designed, I believe, to help overcome and heal these obstacles. A Reiki Principle that you do not like indicates an area in your life that is causing you problems. In the west this is often the principle of Honour Your Parents, Teachers and Elders. You do not solve the problem by leaving out the principle or by changing the principle. You solve the problem by using the principle you do not like every day in your self-treatments.

It is probable that the five Reiki Principles have a connection with the five meditation Buddhas—Aksobhya, Ratnasambhava, Amitabha, Amoghasiddhi and Vairocana.

Just for Today Do Not Anger—
(Buddha Aksobhya-East-Blue)

Buddha Aksobhya promised that on attaining enlightenment he would never get angry again, hence he is known as the Imperturbable Buddha. This seems to indicate that the Reiki Principles act like the promises of a Buddha and if we practice this principle for long enough we, like Buddha Aksobhya, will not get angry but remain imperturbable. This practice should be done on a day to day basis. Making plans to do something for a week, a month, a year or longer often leads to procrastination and failure. "Just for Today" means doing something one day at a time—a more likely method of success. Becoming aware each day of when you are angry, what triggers your anger and what enables you to stop being angry can be done by taking note of how your body reacts to anger. Once you are aware of what makes you angry you can then look at what prevents your anger from arising in the first place. Anger is said to destroy all merit we may have earned.

Just for Today Do Not Worry—
(Buddha Ratnasambhava -South-Yellow)

Buddha Ratnasambhava, the Buddha of Abundance, is known as the Compassionate Giver and his symbol is the "wish-fulfilling jewel". He appears to represent both giving and receiving. In Reiki this principle is sometimes placed first, reflecting Mrs Takata's belief that Westerners are predominantly motivated by money. Worry seems to push away abundance in a person's life. Stop worrying and abundance returns. It takes a great deal of diligence to not allow worry to arise.

A way of dealing with anger or worry is to first become aware of any tension or stress in your body when you worry or get angry, then place your hands where you feel pain or discomfort, so Reiki flows into that area. Next repeat the five Reiki Principles to yourself until your body's response to worry or anger fades away.

Honour Your Parents, Teachers and Elders — *(Buddha Amitabha-West-Red)*

The Reiki Principles handwritten by Mikao Usui in *Reiki, The Legacy of Dr Usui* by Frank Ajava Petter has the third principle as "Show appreciation". *In Living Reiki*, Takata's *Teachings* as told by Fran Brown, it has been extended to "Count your blessings, honour your parents, teachers and neighbours and eat food with gratitude". However, most often the third principle appears as "Honour your parents, teachers and elders". Each of these versions of this principle have in common the ability to rise to that higher part of yourself which can show appreciation, be honourable and count blessings.

Buddha Amitabha, the Buddha of Infinite Light, is the personification of compassion and esoterically represents the Higher Self. He acts as the intermediary between reality and mankind. Amitabha generously forgives every sin—a most appropriate quality for this principle which can be very difficult for some people to accept and which has most often been changed in the west.

This principle is not just about healing your relationship with your parents, teachers and elders but also about healing the attitudes which you have developed because of your experiences with parents, teachers and elders. The attitudes you have towards your parents will crop up again and again in your life whenever you are with someone who reminds you of them or who takes on a parental type role in your life.

Your mother is normally the first person you form a relationship with after birth (even before birth), therefore your mother is the archetype of all relationships in your life. The first experience of anything or any type of relationship becomes the archetype or pattern for all similar experiences or relationships. This principle—Honour your parents, teachers and elders—is also about honouring your archetypes, finding the good within your experiences and relationships so that in the future they will be successful.

Teachers represent your attitudes to learning and also teaching others. They represent your attitudes to people who may have written a book, given classes or just passed on insights and advice which can assist you. If you resent these types of people you will miss out on some valuable help in your life.

Elders represent your attitudes to people in authority in society or who work to ensure the smooth running of society such as police, traffic officers, wardens, social workers and bureaucrats. If your archetypal experiences of these people have resulted in your resenting or resisting such people you will find yourself continually clashing with them. Elders also represent all those messages you give yourself which contain such words as: I must or I must not; I should or I should not; What will my mother, (or father, neighbours, husband, wife, children) think?; and I have to. These words create guilt, inhibitions or rebellion. As you use this principle daily you will find yourself becoming aware of how many times you say "I must" or "I should" and less irritated by your parents, teachers and society's rule-makers.

When we honour someone, we rise up to our higher or honourable self and acknowledge their higher or honourable self. This principle, I believe, also helps us to get in touch with that aspect of ourselves which is "honourable".

Earn Your Living Honestly— *(Buddha Amoghasiddhi-North-Green)*

I believe that this principle lost its true meaning when it was translated from Japanese to English. Because this principle supports the Christian work ethic which prevails in the west, and because Mikao Usui worked with the beggars of Kyoto, most people seem to interpret it as "working for your income honestly".

This particular principle, I think, should be interpreted as *"Earn being alive honestly"* or *"Put Your Studies about Life into Practice, Honestly"*. The north sector of the mandala represents the coldest, toughest time of year. In Chinese philosophy it is said that this is the time when God toils hardest in our lives.

The Buddha Amoghasiddhi personifies putting into practice the things you have studied and learned. He is known as the "Buddha of Infallible Success" because he is a symbol for efficiency and unfailing successfulness.

Show Gratitude to All Living Beings— *(Buddha Vairocana-Centre-White)*

The Buddha Vairocana, Great Sun and primal spiritual essence, is the wheel-turning King who sits at the centre or hub of a circle or wheel. The sun radiates light without any kind of prejudice which enables all living beings to exist on this planet. This principle teaches us to do the same.

Vairocana contains the qualities of the previous four Buddhas. Each one leads to Vairocana, and Vairocana leads to each Buddha. The five Reiki Principles act the same way. Learn not to anger and you will then be able to show gratitude to all living beings. Learn to show gratitude to all living beings and you will find anger cannot arise. Because showing gratitude to all living beings can be difficult to do immediately the first four principles are steps designed to lead us to a point where the fifth principle becomes easier to accept and do.

A few years ago I attended the 99th birthday party of an elderly cousin. I wondered why she had lived so long, why so many people loved her and attended her birthday party. As I listened to her I realised that often during her conversation she would say "Aren't people wonderful? Everyone is so kind". Another comment she frequently made was "I've been so lucky to live through such interesting times." How often do you use statements which honour both yourself and others like these each day? Try them out for a day and see what happens.

Using the Five Reiki Principles

Reiki is a wonderful tool to assist us to heal and make changes in our lives quickly and easily. The only criteria is to use it. The same applies to the Five Reiki Principles; they were meant to be used, not just looked at. Most people just pay lip-service to these wonderful principles. They may frame them, put them up on their wall, then never look at them again or simply put their copy of the principles away in a drawer or cupboard. Apparently, Mikao Usui asked his students to actively work with the Reiki Principles by chanting them morning and evening while holding their hands together in prayer. He asked that we take the principles into our mind, body and spirit.

In Reiki we usually hand out the Reiki Principles during the 1st Degree Class, talk about them a little, give an explanation and then that is it. We do not really give the students a good, practical way of using the Reiki Principles every day. After teaching Reiki for awhile I realised that there needed to be a way to use the Reiki Principles each day. I concluded that the Reiki Principles were "keys" to opening doors within us—doors to communicating with other people in our lives. Many of our "ills" come from how we relate to other people and our relationships with our families. I believe that a very easy way of using the Reiki Principles is to incorporate them into our self treatments. Each of our hand positions (how and where we place our hands) are symbolic and give us subtle messages which can assist the messages of the Reiki Principles.

1. Place your hands over your eyes. Say "Just for Today, do not anger" three times. (What the eyes don't see the heart doesn't grieve about).

2. Place your hands over your temples. Say "Just for Today, do not worry" three times. (The temples are related to the balance of the passive and active sides of the brain, therefore using this principle here indicates balance of thoughts and thinking).

3. Place your hands over the back of your head. Say "Honour your Parents, Teachers and Elders" three times. (This area of the head is related to ancestral memory).

4. Place your hands over your throat. Say "Earn Your Living Honestly" three times. (This is the area of communication).

5. Place your hands over your chest/heart. Say "Show Gratitude to all Living Beings" three times. (This is the area associated with love for other people and with love for ourselves).

Alternatively, you can simply repeat the Five Principles at each of the twelve hand-positions during your daily self-treatment. Using the principles in your self-treatments, or other Reiki treatments, sends them as messages to all the cells of the body.

Buddhists believe in egolessness, which is probably why the Reiki Principles do not have the words "I, me, my, mine or am" in them. This allows these Principles, which are similar to affirmations, to get past the ego. The Buddhists also believe in non-doing so you do not have to, for instance, actively honour your parents, which for some people is almost impossible, all that needs to be done is repeat the Principles each day either as a prayer or as part of your daily Reiki self-treatment. The words go deep into the sub-conscious where they heal the emotions, mental attitudes and relationship archetypes. Enlightenment happens when the principles become second nature to us, when we do them automatically and efficiently without thinking or trying.

Attaining enlightenment means becoming a Buddha. When one of the principles attain enlightenment (when it becomes second nature to us so we do it very well automatically) it means we become a Buddha, for instance: when we simply shrug our shoulders and smile as we see our bus pull away without us on it, instead of getting angry and blaming others for making us late, then we are the Imperturbable Buddha; when we can rise to the honourable part of ourselves (Higher Self) and truly forgive all the sins of our parents, teachers and elders, then we are the Buddha of Compassion; and if we honestly put into practice each step of what we have studied and learned then we are the Buddha of Unfailing Success.

The Five Reiki Principles as a Mandala

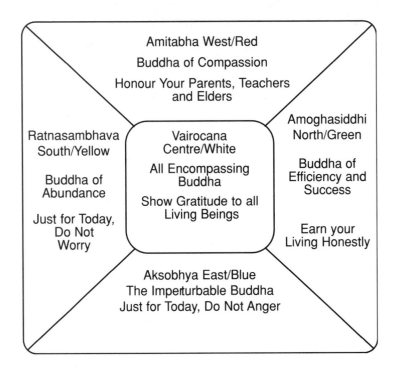

Amitabha West/Red

Buddha of Compassion

Honour Your Parents, Teachers and Elders

Ratnasambhava South/Yellow

Buddha of Abundance

Just for Today, Do Not Worry

Vairocana Centre/White

All Encompassing Buddha

Show Gratitude to all Living Beings

Amoghasiddhi North/Green

Buddha of Efficiency and Success

Earn your Living Honestly

Aksobhya East/Blue
The Imperturbable Buddha
Just for Today, Do Not Anger

Chapter 6

INTRODUCTION TO THE REIKI SYMBOLS

Originally the Reiki symbols were held to be both secret and sacred. These symbols have been said to be sacred because they are energy patterns, while others have said they were sacred because they are used in the Reiki initiations. At the end of my 2nd Degree Reiki class we went through a burning ceremony to destroy all the pieces of paper that I had used during the class. I had to commit the symbols to memory. Like many other Reiki practitioners, the first thing I did when I arrived home from the class was to write down the symbols because I did not entirely trust my memory. Since the publication of books by A J McKenzie-Clay, Kathleen Milner and Diane Stein the shroud of secrecy has been lifted. However, they still remain sacred, although not because they are used in initiations or are energy patterns.

The Reiki symbols are sacred because they represent an aspect of the creative power of the universe which we call God or know as God, and may contain a name of God within them. In ancient times God was never referred to directly. People believed that the name of the creative power of the universe was too sacred to be spoken. For instance, one of the ten commandments of Christianity is "Thou shalt not take the Lord's name in vain." Another was that concepts about the power behind the universe were too great for humanity to comprehend by naming. The language of symbols, such as images, symbols, alphabets, and numbers were used to represent that which is beyond a person's comprehension.

The second level of the mandala represents the mental/emotional level which is viewed as yin or feminine. In the past the life passages of a woman were held to be mysterious, secret and sacred—feminine puberty, menstruation, giving birth, and menopause. The second level of the mandala, which I believe is 2nd Degree Reiki, represents the watersheds of life not just for women but also for men; those times in our lives which have an impact on our psychological make-up; that form our beliefs, opinions, fears, accomplishments, and which ultimately impact on our identity—who we think we are and who we feel we are. This area of ourselves we hold both secret and sacred and is often very securely locked away so that it takes a major disaster to make us change. The 2nd Degree Reiki symbols act as keys to allow us to enter this area of ourselves to create the changes that will heal us, because sometimes the things we have locked into our psychological make-up can be detrimental or harmful to us.

A characteristic of a symbol is that it can express many meanings simultaneously and on different levels. According to Mircea Elaide symbols have three components:

Cosmological—brings to form from the pre-formed or chaos.
Initiation—is used in an initiation rite.
Journey—assists with the spiritual quest in life.
It should be pointed out that Buddhists consider that the pre-formed is not chaos but rather a diamond world of reality where the gods and Buddhas reside.

Within the Reiki community by far the most important aspect of the Reiki symbols is their use in the Reiki initiation, for it is the initiation which activates the flow of the Universal Life Force Energy (Reiki) through the hand chakras and is what basically distinguishes Reiki practitioners from other people who channel energy for healing.

6. Introduction to the Reiki Symbols

Each of the Reiki symbols has a symbol and a name. When using them the symbol is drawn once and the name is spoken or thought three times. There has developed the belief that it is not necessary to use the symbol, that the power is in the name or that the name will suffice. This only applies to the Distance and Master symbols which have symbols that mean the same as their names. The other two symbols are different. They have symbols which are pictures of energy and names which activates that energy. The Mental/Emotional Symbol is a sound-energy symbol. There are many such symbols within Buddhism ie: OM and HUM are also sound-energy symbols. The Mental/Emotional Symbol tells the Reiki vibrational field what sound-energy to work with. The name of the Reiki Mental/Emotional Symbol activates the sound-energy and allows it to work with the healing energy. The symbol and the name have different roles of equal importance, therefore the Power and Mental/Emotional symbols work best when their names and symbols are used together.

Drawing the Reiki Symbols

Because Reiki was re-discovered in Japan the method for drawing the Reiki symbols is based on drawing Chinese and Japanese characters. This method especially applies to the Distance and Reiki Master symbols because they are both made up of Kanji characters. Kanji is a name for the formal written Japanese language. Each Kanji character is meant to appear with the same pattern of strokes each time it is drawn. Therefore the idea that Mrs Takata drew the Kanji characters of the Reiki symbols with different strokes for each of the Reiki Masters she taught must be incorrect—either she did not understand how to write Kanji properly or this belief has come about to justify the different versions of the Kanji Reiki symbols. The following are basic rules for drawing Kanji:

1. Draw the horizontal lines before the vertical lines.
2. Draw the vertical lines from top to bottom.
3. Draw the horizontal lines from left to right.
4. Draw a left stroke before a right stroke.
5. The exception to drawing a left stroke first happens when a right or middle stroke is longer than the left stroke. The longer or "elder" stroke is drawn before any shorter or "younger" stroke.
6. Any strokes that form a 7 shape are drawn as one stroke regardless of whether the vertical part is straight or curved.
7. If you draw a box shape with a stroke inside it then draw the left side of the box first from top to bottom, the top and right side of the box are drawn next as one stroke and before closing the box always draw the stroke inside the square first. The Japanese believe that you cannot put something into a box after it has been sealed, and I agree with them.

The symbols can be written on paper, drawn in the air with your hand or mentally drawn in your mind or with your third eye. Their names can be spoken aloud or thought of quietly in your mind. They can be stepped into, placed in and around your home, placed on your possessions, used during Reiki treatments and Distance Healing, used when meeting people, used at work or wherever you go during the day, and they can be used on each activity you're involved with each day. They are tools which will assist you in all aspects of your life to become more positive, happier and fulfilled.

The Distance and Reiki Master symbols which I have used in this book are Japanese, based on the Kanji characters found in a Japanese/English dictionary. I use the Japanese version of the Reiki symbols because I have found that they give me clarity and understanding of their meanings. I also

6. INTRODUCTION TO THE REIKI SYMBOLS

believe that they would have been the symbols that both Mikao Usui and Chujiro Hayashi used. Because the majority of Reiki Masters in the west do not read Kanji; because the symbols had to be memorised; and because written copies were not allowed to be taken from the class, the Reiki symbols have altered over time; gradually getting more and more out of alignment from the original Kanji characters. The symbols that you use may not look very much like those which appear in this book.

Buddhists and Taoists believe that a symbol is a reflection of our mind, our body, our spirit and that we can improve the condition of our mind, body or spirit by aiming for perfection in the symbols we use. If you have already been initiated to 2nd Degree Reiki you can alter the Distance symbol by simply spending time drawing it until you can remember it and can use it automatically. The most important change you can make is to ensure that all the strokes of the character Nen are contained within your Distance symbol. Those sensitive to energy change will note a powerful and positive shift in the Distance symbol when the Nen has all its strokes. Adding the bottom stroke of the Sho character does little to the energy of the Distance symbol and is, I believe, optional. You can check the energy of your symbols by holding a pendulum above them and observing which way it swings and how wide it swings.

If you have been initiated to 3rd Degree Reiki you can do the same for the Japanese version of the Master symbol. You may find that there will be small shifts and changes within your life, body, mind and spirit as you adjust to the Japanese version of the symbols. There is no need to have a further Reiki attunement/initiation to the Japanese versions, the initiations you received at 2nd and/or 3rd Degree Reiki are enough, all you will be doing is fine-tuning the symbols you

73

learned during those classes. If you have not been attuned to these levels of Reiki the symbols will not work, no matter how often you draw them; you need to attend 1st and 2nd Degree Reiki classes, facilitated by a certified Reiki Teacher, and go through the initiation ceremonies of those degrees to have the 2nd Degree symbols activated, and a 3rd Degree Reiki class to activate the Master symbol.

The Reiki Symbols

The Reiki symbols are sacred symbols because of their interaction with the higher realms of Buddhas or Gods. They are ancient symbols coming from a time when men and women had closer contact with, and a deep belief in, higher beings. As such the names of the symbols should not be abused, profaned or bandied about indiscriminately. When talking to people about the symbols, if you are not teaching their names, then it is best to refer to the symbols in some other way. In the Reiki community this usually means calling them by a number related to the order in which they are taught or by their English term. ie:

Number	Order Taught	English Term
One	1st symbol	Power symbol
Two	2nd symbol	Mental/Emotional symbol
Three	3rd symbol	Distance symbol
Four	4th symbol	Reiki Master symbol

Unless absolutely necessary I will be using the English terms for the Reiki symbols. The Japanese names, I believe, should only be used when working with the symbols. It is also my belief that publishing the Reiki symbols or allowing someone else to see them will not result in any kind of punishment nor any reduction in the power of the symbols. The

6. Introduction to the Reiki Symbols

Reiki symbols are, after all, symbols of healing. They will always move a person towards wholistic wellness. It is a person's feelings of guilt and doubt that punish. The symbols are all displayed in their physical form and sometimes in their seed form in most Buddhist temples and monasteries for all who visit to see.

Using the Reiki Symbols

Some Reiki Masters teach that the symbols should be used in a variety of strictly set orders. My experience has led me to believe that the order in which the symbols are used sets the order of focus for the energy. If the Power symbol is used first then your intention for its use is activated first. If the Mental/Emotional symbol is used first then the first function or focus of Reiki will be mental attitudes and emotional responses to life. Using a Power symbol immediately after the Mental/Emotional symbol ensures that nothing can stop the Metal/Emotional symbol from being effective because it makes the M/E symbol a royal command. If the Distance symbol is used first then the first focus will be to send Reiki to the Ten Directions (Distance Healing). If the Reiki Master symbol is used first then the initial focus of Reiki will be balance, integration and enlightenment. When several symbols are used during a treatment there will be several levels of focus. In the Mental/Emotional technique the first symbol used is the M/E symbol and therefore the first focus of the treatment is to bring harmony and balance to the mental attitudes and emotional responses which are causing imbalances. The second symbol used in this technique is the Power symbol. The secondary focus therefore overcomes (clears away) all negative energies, thoughts and emotions with the receiver being protected throughout the technique and their vibration being raised so that they will feel happier and more positive.

Many Reiki practitioners simply "Let go and Let God" when they are doing Reiki treatments preferring to allow Reiki to determine what is needed for the client. The Reiki system and symbols appear to have originally been designed to allow this to happen. We do not need to know or be consciously aware of why or how Reiki works for it to be effective. However I believe we do need to know why and how Reiki and the symbols work on a conscious level because of our basic need for change and individual expression which tends to be a highlight of western life. Changes have been made within the Reiki system without any understanding of the basic blue-print of Reiki and consequently mistakes and many misconceptions are now to be seen within various Reiki lineages.

Each of the Reiki symbols act as a tool for the journey of life or for any journey you experience, whether it is actual travel to a certain place or the journey of learning a new skill, or experiencing a new relationship, or a Reiki treatment. The Reiki symbols are also keys which allow you to access energetic forces of the universe easily and consistently.

Each symbol has a Japanese name, an interpretation of that name, an English name and a "secret pledge or promise". Although you can use any intent you wish with each symbol as you use it you cannot override the pledge or promise of the symbol. If your intents contradict or do not support a symbol's promise your intents will not be acted upon.

The Reiki symbols are four of the Eight Auspicious Symbols of Buddhism. These four symbols appear on the foot of the Healing Buddha statue at Yakushiji in Japan and, although all eight symbols are depicted on the 51-fold Healing Buddha mandala which appears in *Mystic Art of Ancient Tibet*, the four Reiki symbols are given special places

flanking the east and west gates of the mandala. The four auspicious symbols used by Reiki practitioners are:

Buddhist Symbol	Buddhist Meaning	Reiki Symbol
1. Vajra	Protection/cuts to reality	Power Symbol
2. Conch Shell	Voice of Buddha	Mental/Emotional Symbol
3. Two Fish	Joy of the union of yin and yang	Distance Symbol
	Ability to go anywhere without restraint or constriction.	
4. Vase of Life	Contains spiritual jewels	Master Symbol

The four auspicious symbols not used by Reiki practitioners are:

5. Precious Parasol	Gives protection from evil	
6. Lotus Flower	Emblem of original purity	
7. Knot of Life	Longevity	
8. The Wheel of Life	The Mandala and teachings of Buddhism– spiritual pathway	

The role of Reiki is to transform. To move the practitioner from suffering to wholeness and health. Reiki does not
destroy the ego, but changes your focus away from ego. The
ego can feel jeopardised by the process causing the Reiki
practitioner to give up using Reiki on themselves. The
progress of the transformation that takes place is:

1st Degree	Heals the active energies of the body
2nd Degree	Heals the passive energies of the mind
Power Symbol	Overrides the ego's and soul's blocks and injunctions
Mental/Emotional Symbol	Brings the ego and soul together as one unit
Distance Symbol	Transforms the ego/soul unit into a Buddha/Christ
3rd Degree	Integrates the active/passive energies
Master Symbol	Enables the Buddha/Christ to radiate the light of God and to express itself (enlightenment).

I found it interesting that the four Reiki symbols show a natural progression towards "oneness" which appears to be a nec-

essary part of enlightenment. The central stroke of the Power Symbol is said to represent the axis of the world, that which the world revolves around and which gives the world its balance. The movement of the spiral takes you to the heart or centre of the world which is always looked at as a place of balance. The promise or intent of the Mental/Emotional symbol is "God and Humanity become One" indicating a process of becoming one and telling us what becomes one—our inner God (soul) and our outer Humanity (ego). The first stroke of both the Distance symbol and the Reiki Master symbol is the Japanese/Chinese character for one. The promise of the Distance symbol, which begins with the words "The Buddha in me..." tells us what God and Humanity become. In the Reiki Master symbol the first stroke (one) is part of the word "great" which represents the "the marks of a great man" or those attributes within a person which cause them to act nobly, honourably and with greatness.

Seeding the Symbols

It is said that the Reiki symbols are "seeded" or "planted as seeds" within the initiate during 1st Degree Reiki initiations and are activated at 2nd and 3rd Degree Reiki initiations. This has led some to believe that if they do a lot of Reiki at 1st Degree level the symbols will automatically "grow" so they can use them without having to attend a 2nd Degree Reiki class. This is not how the "seeding" process works. It is not the symbol which "grows" within the initiate but the quality and characteristics of the symbol. To use the symbol in the physical world, as we do in Reiki, the symbol needs to be consciously activated by a Master during an initiation, as happens at 2nd and 3rd Degree Reiki.

OTHER SYMBOLS ASSOCIATED WITH REIKI

Most Reiki practitioners know of and believe that there are only four Reiki symbols—no more, no less. Others have had a vague feeling that there should be more symbols. Consequently more symbols have been added to the Reiki system in the form of Tibetan symbols, Karuna, Tera Mai, Blue Star, Seichem, Seichim, Sekhem, Osho and others with, I believe, little or no understanding of symbols, why they work and what they really do.

A symbol is an archetype—eternally changeless. The clockwise motion represents death and rebirth and therefore change. Many of the symbols which have been added to Reiki are drawn in a clockwise direction and have been through name changes and in some instances, changes to the symbols. For instance the symbols originally known as Sai Baba Healing Symbols have become Tera Mai, Karuna Reiki, Seichem, and Blue Star.

I believe that because the processs of working through the degrees is not understood there has been a search for other symbols and energies which are not needed if we work through the Reiki process properly.

The Tibetan or Fire Symbols

It seems these symbols were the first to be added into the Reiki system. These symbols are drawn clockwise, but when they are drawn counter-clockwise they belong to the mandala for Amitabha, and are symbols for Bodhisattvas. They are not essential for Reiki treatments or Reiki initiations. The Healing Buddha mandala is said to be situated in the east, which in Buddhism is associated with the element of water. The Amitabha mandala is in the west and his element is fire. It has long been considered that fire and water do not mix.

Antahkarana

This symbol is reputed to have been given to Reiki Master Arthur Robertson by Rolf Jensen who claimed it was an ancient Tibetan Master symbol.

The Antahkarana is said to help connect the physical brain with the Higher Self. This is the connection which must develop if we are to grow spiritually. The Buddha Amitabha is said to be a personifica- 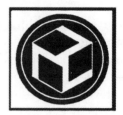 tion of the Higher Self so it is highly likely that the Antahkarana also belongs to the Amitabha mandala. The Antahkarana will activate this connection whenever you are in its presence as well as having a positive affect on your chakras and aura. This symbol always works for good and cannot be misused or cause harm. I have found it works well in meditation, and for healing, but I do not include it in a Reiki treatment. For instance I put it under my mattress when I need extra energy or I will tape it to a part of my body that needs healing when I don't have time to give myself a Reiki treatment. Although not all Reiki lineages use this symbol, its methods of use are usually taught at Reiki Master level.

I believe that the Antahkarana is probably of Chinese origin. In China the square represents Earth and Yin which is dark; the round shape represents Heaven and Yang which is light. The inner circle represents those who live in harmony with the cosmic life and are in communion with the "Great Illuminator" who, in Japan, is known as Dainichi. The three sevens, symbolise the completion of the three levels of a mandala. The cube shape holding the three sevens together represent the eight directions plus above and below. The Antahkarana is in fact a mandala which encloses or encompasses one of the universal energies of life and therefore is a very powerful symbol.

The Johre (Johrei) Symbol = J O K I KEI SHIN

Written in Sosho Japanese—a calligraph which is most often used in Japanese paintings—this symbol consists of four Japanese words; Jo (Pure), Ki (Joy), Kei (Pledged to),

6. INTRODUCTION TO THE REIKI SYMBOLS

Shin (God). Within the Reiki community this symbol has become known as the Johre or Johrei symbol because, according to Kathleen Milner, it was handed out to members of the Johre Society in the USA by a visiting Japanese gentleman who did not tell anyone the name of this symbol or its function. The Johre Society, which owns the copyright for the name Johre/Johrei, has made a statement that it does not want Reiki people using their name for this symbol.

The Jo Ki Kei Shin symbol, in Reiki circles is said to mean "White Light". In *Essential Reiki* and *Reiki and other Rays of Healing* you can see how this symbol, through a lack of understanding the Japanese written language, has been changed into something meaningless.

Kanji, which is the official and formal written language of Japanese, is written in a set stroke-pattern so that a character will appear basically the same each time it is written. Sosho is used in verse or in conjunction with a painting to incorporate a "meaning beyond the words". The writer allows their hand to be guided by intuition or their inner spirit. Therefore, although the characters are written to a general stroke-pattern, they can appear different each time they are written. This means that the Sosho characters of Jo Ki Kei Shin are unique to the moment they were written and contain a "meaning beyond the words" or a spiritual or intuitive message for that moment. The photocopier has made that unique moment available to many.

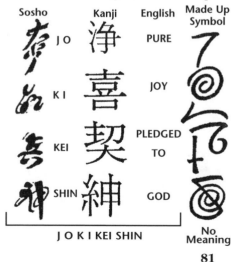

Sosho	Kanji	English	Made Up Symbol
JO	浄	PURE	
KI	喜	JOY	
KEI	契	PLEDGED TO	
SHIN	紳	GOD	
J O K I KEI SHIN			No Meaning

Chapter 7

THUNDERBOLT-IN-THE-HANDS
POWER SYMBOL–1st Symbol of Reiki

Name and Intention

Each of the Reiki symbols has a Japanese name as well as having what appears to be an English translation. The name of the Power symbol is "Cho Ku Rei" which literally translates to *Imperial Command or Royal Edict.* This is the name given to a command or order issued by the Emperor. The English translation which is usually taught in Reiki classes is *"Put the Power of the Universe Here".* This translation is better viewed as the secret intention or promise of the Power symbol rather than the translation of the words "Cho Ku Rei".

The literal translation of the name of the Power symbol leads to the question "Who is the Emperor?" In a family the Emperor is the father or head of a household. In the case of a Chinese Ba Gua the father is represented by the trigram *Heaven* and mother is represented by the trigram *Earth.* Therefore it can be said that the power or energy of the Power Symbol comes from the father or ruler of heaven or the universe. In other words the energy of the Power symbol comes from a higher authority than the person using it and can therefore override all inner mental and emotional commands or injunctions that person may have.

When using the Power symbol the intention *"Put the Power of the Universe Here"* is active yet unspoken and assumed. I believe that the Power symbol becomes more powerful when directed, by stating where you want the power of the universe put. This statement should be clearly made with no attachment to the outcome because the outcome may turn out to be quite different to what you expect. As the power of this symbol comes from the creative force (father) of the universe and is being used in conjunction with the healing energy of the universe (Reiki) results will always be healing and creative in some way.

Origins

The Reiki Power symbol represents the essence or bija of the Vajra. Buddhism took the Vajra from the thunderbolt held by the Hindu god, Indra. This thunderbolt was also held by the Greek god Zeus, the Roman god Jupiter, as well as the early gods of the Assyrians and Babylonians. Even the Christian God has been known to carry a thunderbolt which accounts for the old belief that if you did something to upset God you were liable to be struck by lightning. In Buddhism the Vajra is used as a symbol of wisdom, and having power over illusion and evil spirits (negative thoughts). The Power symbol is the only Reiki symbol which does not come from a written language which may mean that it is older than most written languages.

In the west we have a fear of certain symbols. The swastika, which represents the journey around the four directions, is one symbol which is feared and disliked with intensity. The other symbol is the counter-clockwise spiral. In ancient times the Celtic Druids knew about using symbols and had rituals which involved walking in a counter-clockwise circle. In an effort to destroy the mystery religions of the Druids and others, Christians instigated intense propaganda against such practices and as a consequence the counter-clockwise spiral/circle came to be considered evil when in fact that is not the case. The clockwise movement is the natural movement of our journey through life or any experience we have. The counter-clockwise movement is used to bring into our lives gifts from the universe to be integrated within our centre which will assist us to move through the journey and which will stay with us to use in the future.

One of the stories of the Buddha Sakyamuni is about him receiving a golden bowl. He placed it in a stream. It floated up-stream eventually disappearing into a whirlpool and arriving at the under-water palace of the Black Snake King where it joined the company of other special bowls, striking resonantly against them deep beneath the surface. In *The Buddha* author Michael Pye looks on this as a mythic story about the Buddha. For me this is a story which illustrates the action of the Power symbol—its counter-clockwise direction (up-stream), its spiral (whirlpool), and reaching the heart centre (Snake King). The snake represents wisdom and is to be found at the centre of a Chinese Ba Gua.

The clockwise journey of the mandala represent the journey of the sun from east to west. The counter-clockwise movement appears to represent the journey of the moon (in the Northern Hemisphere) which makes its first appearance in the west, is at its first quarter at the highest point (south) and is a full moon in the east. It begins waning in the west, is in its last quarter at the highest point (south) and wanes just before it reaches the east. In Buddhism the moon is said to represent compassion and benevolence.

In the *I Ching* the clockwise movement is said to be cumulative, to expand with time, and to determine passing events; the opposite, counter-clockwise movement folds and contracts as times goes on, creating the seeds of the future.

It should be noted that the molecules that make up our bodies form themselves in counter-clockwise spirals. A few years ago it was discovered that medicine with molecules built in clockwise spirals causes harmful side-effects to the human body. Thalidomide is an example of this. When it was first tested it had been made as a counter-clockwise spiral

85

and proved to be beneficial, but when it was made in large quantities thalidomide was manufactured using a clockwise spiral (it is easier to build a clockwise molecule) which then had disastrous effects on unborn children. For this reason I do not use the clockwise Power symbol which is taught in Tera Mai, Karuna Reiki, Seichem and Blue Star classes.

In Buddhism the opposite of the Reiki Power symbol would not be a clockwise Power symbol as taught in the above modalities. Because the Power symbol's movement is from the outside into the centre, the opposite would be to move from the centre to the outside, but if drawn from the centre to the outside the essence of the symbol, no longer a gift for us to use in the future, would become a passing event, lost in time.

The Sound of the Symbol

At the centre of the vajra, and therefore the Power symbol, is the sound of HUM—H represents freedom from cause and effect; U represents freedom from arguments; and M represents the groundlessness of the Absolute or Reality.

The Characteristics of the Vajra

The vajra is said to be diamond hard, uncuttable, unbreakable, unburnable, indestructible, like a diamond, therefore in Buddhism the vajra is more often described as a diamond rather than as the thunderbolt it originated from. The Power symbol, as the seed symbol of the vajra, contains the qualities of both the diamond and the thunderbolt. It contains the five wisdoms known as Mirrorlike Wisdom, Wisdom of Sameness, Discriminating Wisdom, Active Wisdom and Wisdom of the Pure Absolute. A vajra initiation is said to sow the seed which grows into unbreakable wisdom. It is also said to contain the five awarenesses and the six perfections.

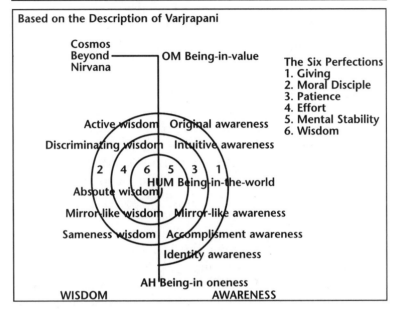

Based on the Description of Varjrapani

Cosmos Beyond Nirvana —— OM Being-in-value

The Six Perfections
1. Giving
2. Moral Disciple
3. Patience
4. Effort
5. Mental Stability
6. Wisdom

Active wisdom — Original awareness

Discriminating wisdom — Intuitive awareness

2 4 6 5 3 1

HUM Being-in-the-world

Absolute wisdom

Mirror-like wisdom — Mirror-like awareness

Sameness wisdom — Accomplisment awareness

Identity awareness

AH Being-in oneness

WISDOM   AWARENESS

The Three Vajras

The vajra can be found on the first, second and third levels of the Healing Buddha's mandala. Having three versions of the vajra in the Healing Buddha mandala indicates that the mandala belongs to Tantric or Vajrayana Buddhism and is also considered a mandala which encompasses or encloses a powerful energy. The Power symbol is used during all the Reiki initiations from 1st Degree Reiki to 3rd Degree Reiki—at both 1st Degree and 3rd Degree it keeps its promises (as described in the Healing Buddha sutras) but is passive or resting; at 2nd Degree it becomes active and alive.

On the first level the vajra is a Yaksha General who promises to protect those who use the energy of the Healing Buddha (Reiki) no matter where they are. This is why people who have received 1st Degree Reiki initiations are protected whenever they use Reiki.

On the second level the vajra becomes the Great Bodhisattva Vajrapani (Thunderbolt-in-the-Hands). Vajrapani is so named because he rises from his Vajra-Wrath (Yaksha General) composure to have the vajra (Power symbol) placed in his hands and to be consecrated (initiated) as the suppressor of all evil. He vows that his command is to be obeyed by all, which explains why the Power symbol is called the Cho Ku Rei (Imperial Command) and is activated during an initiation at 2nd Degree Reiki. As a Bodhisattva (Enlightened Being) Vajrapani works for the happiness and good fortune of all living beings.

On the third level of the mandala the vajra is the Great Mother or Vajradhara who sits in divine meditation and is not active in human affairs, but can still bless and answer all desires, which the Seven Healing Buddhas promise to ensure will be carried out. I think that the first word of the Reiki Master symbol may represent Vajradhara because of the great blessing power which Japanese Buddhists attribute to the character of Dai.

Although some Reiki lineages activate and teach the Power symbol during 1st Degree Reiki classes it still only acts as a passive protector. The student needs to ensure that they also get the Power symbol activated again during their 2nd Degree Reiki class otherwise it will never become an Imperial Command.

The Power symbol brings in energy, knowledge, spiritual help and rewards from the diamond world or the perfect reality. By travelling in a counter-clockwise direction it follows the path of compassion and benevolence. The action of the Power symbol becomes a gift which survives the journey. Once it reaches the centre it is integrated and held there so that it can be used again automatically whenever needed without the necessity of doing the symbol again. However the more times you do a symbol for an event/thing/ thought/feeling the stronger the integration and the more automatic the response will be in future. Eventually you only need to intend the thing, that in the past you used a Power symbol for, and it will manifest. This becomes noticeable when using this symbol to get a car park—one day you forget to do the symbol yet there is a car park in just the right place without consciously having asked for it.

The Chakras

Some Reiki Masters have associated the Power symbol with the chakras. On a physical level the chakras correspond to the endocrine system which sends messages around the body by using hormones. On a spiritual level the chakras act as points in the body where various energetic vibrations from the universe are processed and used by the body. If a chakra is blocked then it becomes difficult to receive the energy, gifts and information that the universe has to offer. Using the Reiki symbols at each of the hand positions can help to unblock the chakras. Below is one way of applying the chakras and endocrine system to the Power symbol.

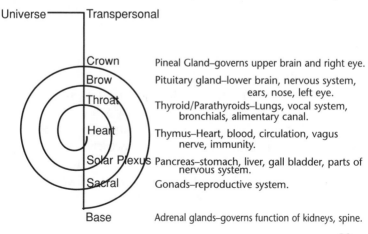

Universe ——— Transpersonal	
Crown	Pineal Gland–governs upper brain and right eye.
Brow	Pituitary gland–lower brain, nervous system, ears, nose, left eye.
Throat	Thyroid/Parathyroids–Lungs, vocal system, bronchials, alimentary canal.
Heart	Thymus–Heart, blood, circulation, vagus nerve, immunity.
Solar Plexus	Pancreas–stomach, liver, gall bladder, parts of nervous system.
Sacral	Gonads–reproductive system.
Base	Adrenal glands–governs function of kidneys, spine.

A Reflection of Ourselves

It appears to me that the symbols can be interpreted in the same way that a writing expert can interpret our handwriting. We do not always write the symbols in exactly the same way each time that we use them. My observation has led me to believe that the symbols often indicate how we are feeling or thinking at the time we draw them—if we are drawing them for ourselves—and if we are drawing them on behalf of someone else then the symbols reflect the feelings and thoughts of the person who is to receive the symbol.

My first realisation of this occurred when I tried sending Distance Healing to a woman who had gone into hospital for observation of her heart condition. I found that I could not mentally draw the Power Symbol—I could not get the spiral to cross the centre stroke. It kept spiralling out to the right side rather than crossing the centre stroke giving me the feeling that the woman was very ill. Later I discovered that her heart condition was worse than I had been led to believe. A day or two after giving her Distance Healing she went into the operating theatre for a triple by-pass operation but while in theatre received a quadruple by-pass.

The Power Symbol seems to reflect our physical condition. You can find these conditions by looking for the places the symbol is not perfect. Draw the Power Symbol several times quickly and then look at the areas which are not quite perfect. If these areas show up in all or most of the symbols you have drawn then it indicates you have a problem there.

The Power Symbol can act as a key which shows where you are blocked. This information becomes obvious when you take note of where the bulges and constrictions occur in the symbol. For instance a constriction between the crown and brow points on the symbol may indicate a block to positive thinking and this may show in the body as sinus. A constriction between the sacral and base points can indicate a block in being positive about creative projects. A large bulge between the base and crown points may indicate wishful thinking or being overly positive about, or placing too much attention on material or sexual matters. You can use the Power symbol to clear away the constriction or to release the bulge. Some further ways of looking at how a Power symbol is drawn are:

Distance between Crown and Transpersonal—if the length of the centre stroke between these two points is short these people are usually very much in touch with their spiritual guides and higher self. If the distance is abnormally long then they are usually unaware of their spiritual guides and higher self. The distance can also indicate how long it takes for goals and affirmations to manifest in their lives. And sometimes it indicates how long it may take someone to recover from a illness.

Difference between the Left and Right Sides of the Spiral—can indicate whether someone is more left (active/wisdom) or right (passive/awareness) brained. Also if one side of the spiral is smaller than the opposite side it can indicate that the person could have physical problems/blocks in that side of their body. Some symbols can look quite narrow or quite fat on both sides of the spiral and this sometimes indicates weight. Fat people often draw "fat" looking spirals.

The Sacral Line drawn below the Base Line—this person is substituting food for sex and can indicate unhappiness with a partner and lack of fulfilment in his/her life—belly can sometimes hang over base chakra area.

The Base Point not in direct line below Sacral Point—this looks like the person has been in a hurry to draw this part of the symbol. These people may have difficulty with waiting for things to manifest, or waiting for people. They may do everything in a rush. Or they can also be avoiding sexual matters—being celibate, have prostrate problem, or have some kind of reproductive problem. It can also indicate bladder problem.

When Distance Between Lines of the Spiral are Narrow—there is a blockage in this area. If, for instance, the blockage is indicated by a narrow space on the right side between the Solar Plexus/Sacral points and the Brow/Throat points then these people have trouble expressing their gut feelings and often dismiss or not follow their hunches. Or if the narrowness is on the left side of the Solar Plexus/Sacral points and the Brow/Throat points then they may have trouble digesting food or information.

Having Difficulty Remembering which Direction to Draw the Symbol—these people have trouble with direction. They can lack a sense of direction. They often don't set goals or have any long term plans in their life. Some retired people have trouble with this because they don't want to look at the end of their life, which is their final goal in this life, due to not resolving their fear of dying.

Not Drawing the Line through the Heart Point—these people may have something wrong with their heart or arteries. They also have difficulty seeing the joy in their lives and find very little enjoyment in anything they do or in their relationships - always complaining.

Distance Between Each Chakra Point Uneven—indicates an imbalance between chakras.

The constrictions in the symbol will also show you where you are not allowing the Life Force Energy to flow properly into your life and where and why you are not accepting the gifts of the universe in your life.

Using the Power Symbol

The Power symbol is perhaps the most versatile of the Reiki symbols. It is easy to use and can be used in many, many ways. More often than not it is used in the physical world outside of ourselves. It can bring us insights, spiritual help, and helps us to move towards excellence and wisdom. Many ways of using the Power symbol are taught during the 2nd Degree Reiki class, where the student is given time to practice the symbol and ask questions about how to use it in their own life. As the student uses the symbol more ways of using it will unfold for them.

The following are a few of the ways I have learned to use the Power symbol.

Burns: If you receive a burn immediately draw a Power symbol, say its name three times and ask that it goes between your skin and whatever is causing the burn to protect you from any further burning. Quickly place the part which is burnt under cold running water until your skin feels cold. Then Reiki the burn with your hands. See a doctor if the burn is a bad one.

Poison: If you swallow any poison, or something very hot, or unpleasant, quickly draw the Power symbol, say its name three times and ask that a thousand Power symbols go into your digestion to protect you from the poison or whatever you have just swallowed. If you have swallowed a poison, contact a doctor immediately.

Travelling: Motors all run at vibrational speeds slower than our normal wakefulness so they often make us feel sleepy. If you find yourself nodding off to sleep or feeling very jet-lagged at the end of a journey place your hands on your solar plexus and mentally draw the Power symbol in front of you, say its name three times and ask it to bring you into balance and harmony immediately with the vibrations of the train, bus, plane or whatever you are travelling in.

The Power Symbol Cleanse: Close your eyes and ask how many Power symbols you need to clear, cleanse and refresh your eyes. When you have been given a number, then: Mentally draw a Power symbol and say its name three times. Then say that you want (say the number you were given) Power symbols to go into your eyes to clear, cleanse and refresh them physically, mentally, emotionally and spiritually. Do the same for other organs in the body such as: sinuses, ears, nose, mouth, throat, bronchial tubes, lungs, gallbladder, spleen, liver, kidneys, pancreas, lymphatic system, and blood. Do this everyday for 21 days. Each day you will notice that the numbers will get lower until one day you will not get any numbers; this means the organ does not need any cleansing for the day.

Pink Happiness: Close your eyes and visualise a large Power symbol, see it filled with soft pink light. Next say the word Happiness three times and see the word going into the spiral and filling the spiral. Then visualise this Power symbol filled with pink light and happiness going into the top of your head and travelling right through your body, into every cell, clearing away all blocks and filling you with beautiful pink light and happiness. Pink is a very healing colour. Alternatively you can ask your intuition for a colour and quality to place in the Power symbol. It is often very interesting just what colour and quality you get. They are always appropriate.

Chapter 8

THE GODDESS
MENTAL/EMOTIONAL SYMBOL - 2nd Symbol of Reiki

Name and Intention

Because the form of the Mental/Emotional symbol is not made up of Kanji characters it is difficult to make a confirmed translation of the words Sei Hei Ki. Although I am told Japanese would not normally read Sei Hei Ki as three separate words but rather as two, Sei Heiki which means habit. For me the translation that best explains the function of this symbol is:

Sei = Sound/Voice; Hei = Together; Ki = Wood/Tree.

Wood and tree are esoteric names for the Healing Buddha. It should be noted that in China the Healing Buddha was also referred to as "King of Healing Tree Buddha" and "Victorious Healing Tree Buddha". This is because the Healing Buddha's mandala is situated in the eastern sector of a Buddha-Star System and the element associated with the eastern direction in China is wood or tree.

The word "sound" can esoterically represent the Buddhist deity Avalokitesvara who appears on the second level of the Healing Buddha mandala and who is well known as the Bodhisattva of Compassion. Therefore, based on my translation above, the esoteric meaning of Sei Hei Ki would be:

Compassion together with Healing

The intention or promise of this symbol is *"God and Humanity Become One"* which aims at bringing the soul or spiritual essence (God) within us and our ego (humanity) into one unit. This is sometimes expressed as bringing the body (temple of God) and the mind (consciousness/ego) into harmony so that they work together as one unit. When God and

Humanity within us becomes one then we can become "one" with the God or Power of the Universe encompassed within the symbol. Compassion and the healing power of Reiki would appear to be the two elements that can achieve this melding of soul/spirit and ego.

Origin

The Mental/Emotional symbol seems to have evolved from a letter of the Gupta alphabet (an early form of Sanskrit) which represents the sound "áh". The first letter of many alphabets has been used as a mystic symbol for the ultimate beginning or creation of the universe and for the creative power which brought the

Long Ah Sound from Gupta Alphabet

Gupta - Language of the First Kings to Patronise Buddhism

cosmos into being. Hence many of the names of God contain this sound—Yahweh, Jehovah, Allah, Ra, Baal, Ahura Mazda, Mab, Atman, etc. The Buddhists recognise the five forms of the sound of "a" as sacred sounds—*a, á, am, ah, áh* which can be illustrated as a mandala. I-hsing, an ancient Buddhist translator said that the last áh pervades everywhere and satisfies all kinds of human desires.

The use of the *Ah* sound goes back to the earliest period of Indian religion, beyond the time when Indian Buddhism was founded over 2,500 years ago. The letter for Ah may be up to 4,000 years old and the belief that it is the subtle body of a god is said to have probably started in the second century BC, by someone called Patanjali.

96

8. THE GODDESS

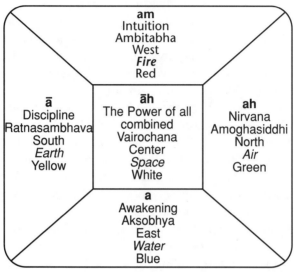

	am Intuition Ambitabha West *Fire* Red	
ā Discipline Ratnasambhava South *Earth* Yellow	**āh** The Power of all combined Vairochana Center *Space* White	**ah** Nirvana Amoghasiddhi North *Air* Green
	a Awakening Aksobhya East *Water* Blue	

The sounds of A appear to be very primal, probably coming from a time when sounds rather than language were used by humans. They are sounds which also convey information, for instance the long A sound which appears in the south section of the above mandala is the sound mothers often use to growl or warn small children. The long ah at the centre of the mandala is the sound we say when we are satisfied with something—"*Aaaah*" or when we say the sound of "Ah" while letting out a long breath.

The Sei Hei Ki is a "seed" or bija symbol representing the quality within the power of the universe which enables a person to rise to a higher state of consciousness and to achieve the necessary state of mind to attain "Enlightenment" or "Oneness with God". The quality the Sei Hei Ki appears to be compassion.

All the vowels of Sanskrit are considered to be female or in other words the passive expression of God. Therefore the God that this symbol represents must appear in the passive section of the Healing Buddha mandala and this is where Avalokitesvara, known to have feminine versions, sits. These feminine versions known as Pandra in India, Kwan Yin in China, Tara in Tibet, and Kwannon in Japan often have various representations associated with colour. The position of *Ah* at the centre of the mandala above indicates that the deity embodied within the Mental/Emotional symbol is Pandravasini (which in Sanscrit means Pandra Clad in White), Pai-i Kwan Yin (Kwan Yin Clad in White) or White Tara. Avalokitesvara's name, "Observer (*passive action*) of the Cries (*sounds*) of the World", also indicates his/her association with this symbol. The Mental/Emotional symbol is the most passive of the Reiki symbols.

Alexander Soper in *Literary Evidence for Early Buddhist Art in China*, suggests that Avalokitesvara originates from an intermingling of Persia's Mithra and India's Siva. Avalokitesvara is said to save people from fire, water, demons, fetters and the sword. I would like to suggest that these dangers are related to the various mandalas that Avalokitesvara appears in: fire = Amitabha mandala; water = Healing Buddha mandala; demons = Vidya mandala; fetters = Maitreya mandala; and the sword = Sakyamuni mandala.

Avalokitesvara is said to be able to see and hear all suffering in the world and has vowed to save all beings with great compassion and consequently he is often depicted with a thousand arms and a thousand eyes to enable him to see all and help all. Avalokitesvara is said to manifest in many forms, including human form with the Mental/Emotional symbol being just one of the forms. As Kwan Yin he is the deity that women pray to when they want to have a son. It is sometimes noted within Reiki groups how many women fall pregnant after learning Reiki. Mrs Takata recommended Reiki treatments for women wanting to have a baby.

8. THE GODDESS

Lotus-in-the-Hands

Avalokitesvara is also known as Padmapani which means Lotus (Padma) in-the-hands (pani). This name indicates that like Vajrapani his symbol is also placed in the hands during an initiation. In Buddhism this is usually done by placing a bell into the hands of the initiate. Because pani is plural it appears the symbol is activated in both hands during an initiation.

Key to the Guardian

When I first learned 2nd Degree Reiki I was told by my Master that the Mental/Emotional symbol was a key for getting past the "dragon at the gate", and that it was supposed to look like a dragon that guards the entrance to a temple. My interpretation of the Bodhisattva families is that each family is like an enclosed building which contains a group of associated or family-like thoughts and emotions. At the entrance to this family stands a Doorman who lets in or keeps out other associated thoughts or emotions, followed by a Guardian who also determines which thought or emotions can enter the family. Some of the members of the family do not always get along. You will know this when you find yourself sabotaging things that you really want to do such as; giving up smoking, losing weight, saving money, learning a new skill, or sabotaging your relationships so that they are often unhappy or unrewarding. For instance our family of money thoughts can contain thoughts of both poverty and wealth. We can have difficulty changing our thoughts and attitudes—we will make some progress because we pass the Doorman but we then find ourselves going no further because we didn't get passed the Guardian.

It appears to me that Reiki gets us past the Doormen and this is done when we use the Hand Positions and the Five

Reiki Principles. The Mental/Emotional symbol gets us past the Guardian by first healing the Guardian. When followed by the Power symbol the whole process of healing (making our thoughts work for our highest benefit) becomes a royal command which must be obeyed and overcomes any negative (evil) thoughts, attitudes, or emotions that are preventing the Guardian from working for our highest good. The Mental/Emotional symbol is like a master key which opens every room in a house—in other words it can open/get past/heal all Guardians, not just a specific one.

My Interpretation of the Mental/Emotional Symbol

By looking at the Mental/Emotional symbol as a head you will begin to see how and when to use the symbol.

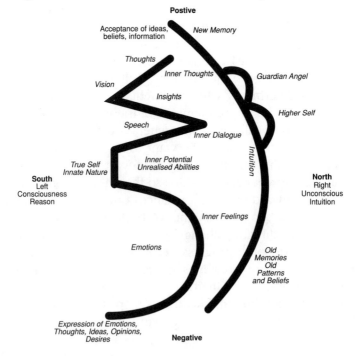

8. The Goddess

The outside of the first stroke of this symbol represents our outward expression of our thoughts, speech and emotions. The only straight part of the symbol (which would remain in the same place if you were to swivel the symbol around) represents our True Self—our essence which we brought with us into this lifetime and to which we add our integrated experiences.

Thoughts. The length of this stroke indicates the length of time spent thinking about something—a very long line can indicate someone who worries a lot. A very short line indicates someone who is thoughtless, speaks without thinking or is lacking in tact.

Vision. Your observation of the world around you. Seeing clearly the symbols and signs that the universe sends us to help us understand ourselves better by seeing those aspects of yourself which are reflected in others. Takes notice of what is happening.

Speech. Short lines indicate short, clipped speech; longer lines indicate a slower way of talking. A narrow gap indicates a "closed mouth" person or someone who doesn't speak often. A large gap indicates a very talkative person. Not much room between the point created by these lines and the intuition area indicates someone who can "talk on their feet" or "off the top of their head" easily often not really knowing from where they have received the information they are passing on.

True Self. This is the only vertical stroke in the whole symbol and can be seen to be that point within us that cannot change—our essence, our innate nature, or some would say our soul, the part of us which is truly ourselves. The symbol will endeavour to bring in what is needed for us to be true to ourselves and to enable us to express our innate

101

nature. A long stroke here can indicate some stubbornness, intractability or determination. If this stroke is not drawn at all it can indicate that the person is completely out of touch with their true self.

Emotions. The size and depth of this stroke indicates how emotional a person is. A minimal curve equates to shallow emotions; a large curve to deeply felt emotions. If this curve is disproportionate to the rest of the symbol the person is very focused on their emotions and can be disproportionately emotional.

CENTRE OF SYMBOL

In Eastern philosophy space is important. When using mudras, the space created by the way hands and fingers are held is as important as the hand or fingers used. In a home the space between the walls is important because it is the area where we live. The space in the middle of the Mental/Emotional symbol represents what is going on inside us, in our thoughts and feelings. An important part of becoming balanced is to bring our outer expression into agreement with our inner thoughts and feelings. Often we will say something that is completely different to what we think. Have you ever said, "I can't do that, I'm not feeling very well," when you really mean, *"I hate helping, but I don't want anyone to think I'm a dreadful person for not helping so I am pretending to be sick"*. The body is always honest and if you spend a large amount of your time saying one thing while thinking another your body will begin to bring you to a point of honesty—especially if you use sickness as an excuse—eventually you will really become sick, often just when you don't want to.

If this area is large and fat looking with a very narrow gap at the bottom, then the person holds back their feelings and thoughts. Many of the difficulties in their relationships with other people will be caused by being unable or unwilling to communicate with others.

Acceptance of Ideas, Beliefs and Information A large gap here indicates taking in everything you see, hear, read, etc without making any judgements or without analysing— this can mean you can be susceptible to suggestion. A very narrow gap indicates you are judgmental and analyse everything you see, hear, read, etc before accepting the information. We are more likely to take in information when it is presented to us in a very positive manner as this area of the symbol is situated at the positive polarity.

Inner Thoughts, Dialogue, Feelings Everything that you take in, information, beliefs and ideas, must run the gauntlet of your inner thoughts, dialogue and feelings. Everyone does this processing—some spend a long time at it and the symbol can be very long and narrow. Others go through this processing very quickly, almost as if they haven't thought about it very much which can mean that they understand basic principles and how to apply them easily or they can be rather thoughtless—not spending enough time integrating information, beliefs or ideas so that they appear to parrot someone else's ideas. Their symbol can be quite short or squat looking.

Insights These are the ideas and thoughts which are gained during the processing of your inner thoughts and dialogue. Some can arrive suddenly without seeming to have any back-up information and can be considered a "leap in imagination". These insights or leaps are often when we argue with ourselves by refusing to acknowledge the information received in this way. I call this "arguing with your Guardian Angel".

Inner Potential, Unrealised abilities We all have potential and special abilities. Many people believe that these are the positive results of previous lives. Scientists have found that memories of things learned by a parent can be passed on to a child through the memories contained in genes. This can mean that the child will be good at whatever the parent learned before they were conceived. The child will still need to learn and practice but in the end will probably exceed their parent's ability because they have the added advantage of inheriting the essence of the ability from that parent. Because there seems to be a deep need to protect and nurture them, expressing our inner potential and unrealised abilities can often be a painful process consequently they often end up as lost dreams and wishful thinking. Using the Mental/Emotional symbol can help to bring these dreams to expression in a way that is safe while at the same time being just a little bit adventuresome and exciting.

Expression of emotions, thoughts, ideas, opinions, desires This gap shows how inner thoughts, dialogue and feelings as well as opinions and desires are expressed. A large gap indicates someone who will tell "their whole life story" within a short time of meeting you. Or alternatively this is someone who does a lot of talking such as a teacher, salesperson or radio announcer. A small gap indicates someone who may have difficulty expressing their feelings, thoughts and opinions. We need to be aware of how we are expressing ourselves because this area of the symbol in situated at the negative polarity. It is easier to express our thoughts, ideas and opinions in a negative manner than it is to express them in a positive way. Learning to express ourselves in a balanced way enables us to express our True Self.

INNER SIDE OF THE SECOND STROKE

This is the area of intuition and those things which are at the back of the mind just waiting to come into your awareness. It is the subconscious area of the mind.

8. The Goddess

Intuition. We all have some experience of intuition. Some people dismiss the gut-feelings, the little voice in their heads, or thoughts that seem to come from out of nowhere, while others will argue with them. Intuition comes from the subconscious which, although it cannot express itself with language like the conscious mind, is equally as useful and intelligent. It will express itself in images, feelings, music, dreams and old memories.

Outside the Second Stroke

This area appears to express memory, both old and new. These memories can be used by the subconscious mind to indicate when a person is repeating an old pattern which does not benefit them by triggering that memory and any painful feelings around them. The Mental/Emotional symbol will also bring up painful memories which need observing and healing.

New Memories. This area of the symbol indicates the ability to learn, to remember new information, and to develop talents which require learning and practice. A short stroke here indicates that the person has some difficulty learning, while a long stroke shows that the person finds learning very easy. I have seen someone who had no new memory ability (because of virus damage) being unable to draw this part of the Mental/Emotional symbol no matter how many times he drew the symbol and even though he had a copy of the symbol in front of him to make copying easy. We are more likely to learn something new when it is presented in a positive way because this part of the symbol is situated at the positive polarity.

Old Memories, Patterns, and Beliefs. If this area of the symbol is short then the person will have little interest in the past or they have an area of their past that they have blotted out. A long stoke indicates a long memory—students in their fifties or sixties often have a longer stroke here than people in their teens or early twenties. It can also indicate the ability to hold on to old grudges. Old memories, patterns and beliefs can act as a trigger for deeply held feelings and emotions. The intuition can utilise old memories to point to something similar happening in your present life or to give you a solution to a problem.

THE TWO BUMPS AT THE BACK OF THE SYMBOL

These two half circles indicate the points where we connect with the universe and is known as the super-consciousness. The two half circles mean that they are drawn firstly moving away from the subconscious area of the symbol and then moving towards it, indicating that there is a two-way movement between ourselves and the universe.

Higher Self/Guardian Angel. These strokes on the symbol represent our connection with the higher energies/beings of the universe. It's through this connection that we receive "help from heaven" usually passed to us through our intituion. If these strokes are placed opposite the inner thought area then intuition will come through more strongly as visions and thoughts. If they are opposite the speech area then you may have an ability to channel information or to receive intuitive thoughts through inner dialogue. If these strokes appear lower down then intuition will be experienced more strongly as feelings and hunches or may be given through old memories. When opposite the unrealised abilities area the intuition may be expressed through music, song, poetry or art.

Using the Mental/Emotional Symbol

Initially I was taught that the Mental/Emotional symbol could only be used during the Mental/Emotional Technique. By understanding the information contained within the Mental/Emotional symbol it becomes clear that this symbol can also be used for all those aspects shown on the above symbol.

> **MENTAL**: *Inner thoughts; insights; acceptance of information; memories.*
> **COMMUNICATION:** *Speech; expression of thoughts and ideas.*
> **EMOTIONS**: *Feelings; emotions; opinions, desires, old patterns, beliefs.*
> **SPIRITUAL**: *Intuition; interaction with guides and higher self; true self and potentials.*

When needing help with any of the above, mentally state your intention three times then draw the Mental/Emotional symbol and say its name three times. For example:

INTENTION	MENTAL/EMOTIONAL SYMBOL
Bring my inner thoughts and feelings into perfect harmony	Draw once, say name 3 times.
Bring my outer speech and inner thoughts into perfect harmony	Draw once, say name 3 times.
Allow me to express myself confidently and truthfully	Draw once, say name 3 times.
Allow my intuition to provide me with clear answers	Draw once, say name 3 times.
Allow me to retain the information in this book I am about to read	Place hands on book then draw symbol once over book say symbol's name 3 times.

The symbol will harmonise our mental processes with our emotional responses, allowing us to say what we mean and mean what we say. It will bring calmness and clarity to our thoughts and emotions. Harmony will also be brought to the expression of our true self and unexpressed potentials. It finds the balance point between our extremes of positive and negative on the mental and emotional level and also brings more harmony to the left (conscious–ego) and right (sub-conscious–soul) sides of our brain.

The Mental/Emotional Technique

The Mental/Emotional technique is taught and practiced during the 2nd Degree Reiki class. This technique is used for those people who need help with mental and emotional problems. It becomes really effective when the hand position is held for fifteen minutes or more. After about five minutes the client may get restless and ask you to stop. Negotiate with them for an extra couple of minutes. After six to seven minutes the client will settle down and allow you to treat them for a long as you want. This technique is best used at the beginning of a counselling session as it allows the problems which are upsetting or holding back the client to come to the surface and be expressed. You can repeat this technique during the session if the client becomes distressed. The Mental/Emotional technique will eventually bring the client a sense of peace and allow them to find a way of solving and letting go of whatever has upset them.

Reiki and Sound

Because I believe the name of the Mental/Emotional symbol can mean "Sound together with Healing" I have used this symbol in the following way.

8. THE GODDESS

1. Place your hands over the area of the body that needs healing. Close your eyes and ask if there is a sound that will help with healing this area. If the answer is yes, ask what sound to use. (I usually get a number. I then choose the letter of the alphabet which corresponds with the number ie: 1 = a; 13 = m; 22 = v, etc).
2. Next draw the Mental/Emotional symbol over the area that needs healing, then place your hands on it and say the M/E symbol's name three times.
3. Breathe in, then on the out breath sing the letter of the alphabet you have been given. Visualise or intend that the vibration of the sound going out through your hands into your client. If you are shy about singing aloud you can sing the sound mentally - not quite so effective but it still works. Keep singing the sound for 3 to 5 minute or until you feel you should stop.
4. When you finish draw a Power symbol over the area before taking your hands away.

Chapter 9

DISTANCE HEALING
DISTANCE SYMBOL–3rd Symbol of Reiki

The Distance symbol is very important in Reiki because this is the symbol which enables Reiki practitioners to send healing energy across distance and time. Often this is the only use made of this symbol, yet it should always be remembered that symbols can have a number of functions.

The Distance symbol is a series of Kanji characters which overlap and combine to form a heart-mantra. In Buddhism it is said that when syllables or characters overlap there is greater power which permeates your whole body with a sense of clarity, purity and higher awareness. Japanese do not normally overlap their written characters in the way that the characters within the Distance symbol overlap and they therefore find this arrangement of characters difficult to comprehend. Overlapping of Chinese characters was done by early Buddhists and Taoists in China to create magical formulas. Tibetan Buddhists also overlapped Sanscrit letters to create powerful syllables used in mantras. This overlapping of the characters within the Distance symbol indicates that it is both powerful and magical.

Of all the 2nd Degree symbols the Distance symbol is most obviously identifiable as Japanese. A quick look in a Japanese-English dictionary of Japanese characters will enable you to find some explanation of the meaning for this symbol. However, if you do not understand that the Distance symbol has been put together as a heart-mantra then you will become confused as you progress with your research until you realise the Japanese characters in this symbol overlap. Because the symbol is sacred and esoteric it has been devel-

111

oped so that only those who know about it will fully understand it.

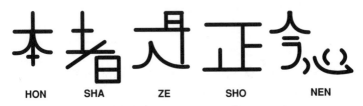

HON   SHA   ZE   SHO   NEN

How and Where the Distance Symbol Overlaps

(The bold strokes relate to the name beside it)

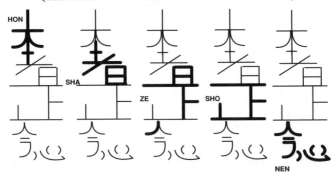

After researching this symbol I chose to use
the version shown above, although I cannot say
that it is the correct version. Mrs Takata left four
strokes out of her verson of the Distance symbol
and there is one stroke (the right curved stroke of
Ze) left out of the Distance symbol I use. It should
be noted that the second curved stroke of Ze is
not the same as the second stroke of Nen.

Mrs. Takata's
Distance Symbol

Name and Intention

A literal translation of the symbol's name is: *This (Hon)
Person (Sha) Rightly/Justly (Ze) Corrects/Adjusts (Sho)
Thoughts/Feelings/Cares/Concerns/Desires (Nen).* The promise

or intention of this symbol is *"The Buddha in me reaches out to the Buddha in you to promote Enlightenment and Peace"*. The Distance symbol recognises that each one of us equally contains the spark of God or the potential of Buddhahood. It also indicates that once we recognise that each of us is a part of God then our relationships can be conducted in enlightenment and peace.

The Bodhisattva of the Distance Symbol

The Distance symbol appears to be the bija or seed symbol for Manjushri (Gentle Glory), who can be found alongside Avalokitesvara in the eastern segment of the second level of the Healing Buddha mandala, and is the Bodhisattva who personifies wisdom and intellect. He is usually depicted carrying the sword of wisdom and a book, said to be the Prajnaparamita (Wisdom of Perfection) sutra. The Distance symbol can also be interpreted as Book (Hon) Person (Sha) Righteously (Ze) Corrects (Sho) Thoughts (Nen), signalling the Distance symbol's association with Manjushri.

Although Manjushri, known as Monju in Japan, abides in the east (female), is seen standing on the left (female) side of Buddha Sakyamuni, and is known as the father and mother of multitudes of Buddhas pointing to an association with the Great Mother, he is almost never depicted as a woman but is usually seen as an ever-young, celebate prince. Celebacy is often used in Buddhism to depict non-duality or the point where female and male are in complete balance and cannot be distinguished as either female or male.

Manjushri also has an ancient association with the ocean which may explain why a pair of fish are used to depict the Distance symbol on the foot of the Healing Buddha at Yakushiji. His status as a "consecrated heir of the Buddha" points to an involvement with initiations or consecrations.

Manjushri's text was translated into Chinese by the end of the third century AD, which could mean the Distance symbol may have made its first appearance around that time.

Manjushri is sometimes depicted holding a bow and five arrows said to represent five syllables making it interesting to note that the Distance symbol is made up of five words which when overlapped, as they do in the symbol, give the appearance of five syllables in one word or character. The flight of the arrows, which are said to hit various parts of the body, is a good metaphor for Distance Healing. Another such metaphor can be seen in Manjushri's duty to perserve the true faith of enlightenment in the interval between two Buddhas; in other words, he acts as the bridge when the Buddha in me reaches out to the Buddha in you. Some of the vows that Manjushri has made include:

1. Always acting for the benefit of sentient beings without greed, miserliness or resentfulness.
2. Observing complete morality and perfect purity.
3. Causes his name to be known throughout the ten directions.
4. Never tries or wishes to attain a rapid, self-seeking enlightenment, but continues to benefit all sentient beings until the end of the future.

Immense benefits are said to arise from seeing an image of Manjushri and also from saying his name. According to the Healing Buddha sutra, because of Manjushri's great thoughts of compassion and pity, by his request, sentient beings will obtain joy and peace from karmic fetters, suffering and afflictions.

Characters with the Distance Symbol

The true meaning of esoteric is not secret knowledge but in fact "hidden knowledge". Many of us, as children, have played games where we have searched for hidden pictures within a picture, or hidden words within a word. You can do the same with the Distance symbol, although Japanese would not read the symbol in this way, the amazing thing is that when you discover the hidden words within this symbol they tell you how this symbol works.

At all times use the complete Distance symbol. The various symbols within it are not meant to be used on their own. Together, as the Distance symbol, they reach a high metaphysical level which activates the archetypal realms of consciousness.

**Symbol Within
The Distance Symbol**   **Meaning**

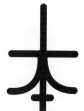

HON = This, Book, True, Root
MOTO = Origin, Basis, Capital (Money)
Buddbist: Radical; fundamental;
original; one's own principle.

This symbol within the Distance symbol has a twofold purpose. Firstly it represents Manjushri and also the other Bodhisattvas who appear in the Healing Buddha's mandala holding a book, consequently I think the Distance symbol could be used wherever the symbol of a book is depicted in that mandala. Secondly it indicates that the Distance symbol can be used to connect with the origins or root of a problem or event. It can also be used to connect with the truth of a problem or event or with our own inner truth. The Distance symbol can also be used to connect with the cause of money problems or to find original ways to generate more money in your life.

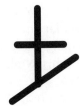

SAI = Ability, Wit, Talents, Intelligence

This character indicates that the Distance symbol can be used to discover and connect with your latent, inner potentials and unrealised abilities. The distance symbol can assist you when learning something new or when you are developing one of your talents.

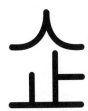

KUWADATSU = To plan, to project

Although the two parts of this character are not shown together within the Distance symbol this character can be found and does indicate a function of the Distance symbol. The Distance symbol can be used to send Reiki and the Reiki symbols to any plans you have for the future. It can also project Reiki and the Reiki symbols into the future for any event. Manjushri's promise to help sentient beings until the end of the future indicates that the symbol works until all aspects of the event are complete which may take a longer than you anticipated.

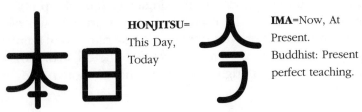

HONJITSU= This Day, Today

IMA=Now, At Present. Buddhist: Present perfect teaching.

Each of the Reiki symbols begins working as soon as you have completed drawing it. Often the reason the symbols don't appear to work is because of the time it can take to get everything into its right sequence and right place. This is especially so when the Distance symbol is used to send energy to an event in the future. The Buddhist interpretation of Ima indicates that the Distance symbol could be used by Reiki Teachers to help them when teaching a Reiki class.

 DO–Earth, Soil, Ground. Buddhist: Earth, locality, local.

The Distance symbol can be used to send Reiki to any locality. It can also be used to ground or earth a person by drawing it on the soles of the feet. Or to send Reiki into the soil or for the planet Earth.

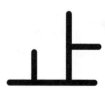 **TOMERU**–to stop, hold up, fasten. Buddhist: Putting to rest the active mind; the mind centred; getting rid of distraction; ceasing to do evil; when the mind is seeing clearly;

This character is why the Distance symbol can be used to hold the other Reiki symbols in one place for a particular period of time, such as on your bed, car, in doorways and windows, on a showerhead, etc. When wanting to hold symbols in a certain place use the Distance symbol last and state how long you want the symbols to remain in that place.

The Buddhist meaning indicates that the Distance symbol can be used during meditation to centre and still the mind

117

and let go of distractions. This character means that the mind will cease to do evil (have negative thoughts) while the Distance symbol is being used and is another reason why Distance Healing cannot be used for evil or negative intent.

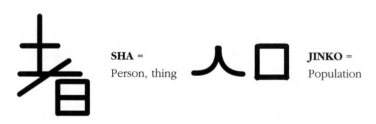

SHO = Best, Far Better, Superior

AGERU = to raise, Increase, Give

I like seeing this character as part of the Distance symbol, confirming that the Distance symbol is always working for the highest good. Mrs Takata left the bottom horizontal stroke out of this part of the Distance symbol when she drew it. Because of the meanings of this character (Sho) and the previous character (Tomeru) I chose to include it in the Distance symbol I use.

SHA = Person, thing

JINKO = Population

These two symbols indicate that Reiki can be sent to one person, an object/event, or to a large group of people. The energy does not decrease if it is sent to a group of people no matter how large the group. Each person in the group will receive the amount of energy they need at that time. When sending to an event Reiki will go to all those people who will be involved in that event.

SHIN = Heart, Feelings. *Buddhist*: The heart, mind, soul; the source of mental activity; totality of mind. *Zen*: a person's powers of consciousness, mind, heart, spirit; absolute reality; self-nature or true nature.

This character indicates that the Distance symbol connects from heart to heart or from the Buddha in me to the Buddha in you. It also indicates that the Distance symbol can be used to connect with feelings, enabling us to connect with those feelings that need to be healed. It helps us to send out a "resonance" to the universe, the future, or to someone who needs it which will allow them to "resonate" or be in tune with their true nature or essence.

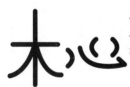

Buddhist: (name not given in Chinese Buddhist Dictionary–just symbol and meaning): The original heart; or mind; one's own heart.

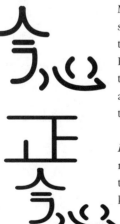

NEN = Thoughts/Feelings/Cares/Concerns. Zen: Mind directed to the moment; attention; intensive, concentrated, nodualistic or non-judgmental thought. *Buddhist:* (In Sanscrit = Smriti) Recollection, memory, to think on; reflect; a thought; a movement; tradition; mindfulness of all mental and physical activities; Smriti is said to be free from falsifying influences.

Buddhist: (In Sanskrit = Sanyak-smtri) Correct remembrance or memory, which retains the true and excludes the false; benevolence and kindness.

119

These three sets of characters indicate that the Distance symbol is a tool to assist the process of meditation. They indicate that the Distance symbol could be used to assist with the recovery of memories, ensuring that those memories brought forward are true and not wishful thinking. Most importantly these characters show that the Distance symbol ensures that Distance Healing is sent with kindness and benevolence from the heart without false concepts.

Cosmology of the Distance Symbol

Also found within the Distance symbol are characters which can esoterically refer to enlightened beings. They assist in taking the energy from the person sending it to the person or persons receiving it. They enable the symbol to work across both time and space/place as well as ensuring that the energy has the "knowingness" or knowledge of what is needed to heal the person or event.

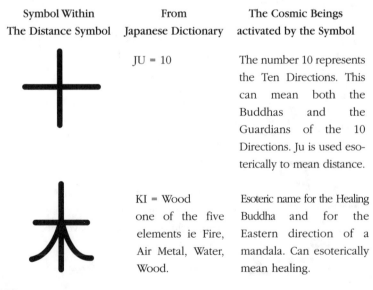

Symbol Within The Distance Symbol	From Japanese Dictionary	The Cosmic Beings activated by the Symbol
	JU = 10	The number 10 represents the Ten Directions. This can mean both the Buddhas and the Guardians of the 10 Directions. Ju is used esoterically to mean distance.
	KI = Wood one of the five elements ie Fire, Air Metal, Water, Wood.	Esoteric name for the Healing Buddha and for the Eastern direction of a mandala. Can esoterically mean healing.

9. DISTANCE HEALING

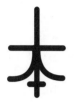

HON = Book

The Bodhisattvas Manjusri (East), Nagavrksa (South); Darsaniya (West) each has a book symbol representing knowledge and wisdom.

According to the Healing Buddha sutra Manjushri promises to carry the name of the Healing Buddha to all sentient beings and whisper it to them. He has also promised to cause his name to be known throughout the ten directions. The character of Hon appears to incorporate the idea of these promises.

NICHI = Sun = time

This symbol represents time hence the 12 Yaksha Generals who promise to protect no matter where someone lives.

These bijas within the Distance symbol basically describe the action of the symbol. The healing energy is sent out to people (Buddhas of the Ten Directions) with wisdom (enlightenment) ensuring that all healing takes place at the right time and right place. The esoteric meanings of the first two characters Ju and Ki, name the symbol—Distance Healing.

Where the Kanji characters are placed within the Distance Symbol seem to also indicate when to use the symbol. Because the first two characters are Ju (distance) and Ki (healing) the Distance Symbol is used first when sending Distance Healing. Because the Kanji character for Tomeru, which means to hold or fasten, is near the end of the Distance Symbol it indicates that the Distance Symbol should be used last when wanting to hold the other Reiki symbols in a particular place or time.

The Distance Healing Technique

In quantum physics it is said that quantum waves can go both forward and backward in time. For an event to take place there must be two events; the present event which is called a stimulating event and a future event which is called the responding event. Each event sends out a quantum wave which acts like a "handshake across time". The stimulating event sends a quantum wave into the future and the responding event sends a quantum wave from the future to the present. If the two waves have a similar resonance then the future event will be observable ie: it will "happen". The Distance symbol enables us to make that "handshake" and also find the responding event that resonates the best for us easily. The symbol contains within it elements for time, the future and the present; and also the resonance of thoughts and feelings, and a "beat"—our heart beat which is symbolised within the Nen character.

The Reiki technique of Distance Healing is very easy and simple. However, for it to work effectively you need to have been initiated to the Reiki symbols by a certified Reiki Master. Some 1st Degree Reiki practitioners have tried learning the symbols from a book. They found that simply learning how to draw the symbols was not enough. They had to attend a 2nd Degree Reiki class to have the Reiki symbols activated. At 1st Degree Reiki the symbols are said to be in repose or resting but are "awakened" or activated during a 2nd Degree Reiki initiation. Most Reiki Teachers will teach several ways of using the Distance Healing technique during a 2nd Degree Reiki class. The student can then choose which method they prefer working with.

The Distance symbol has been described as both a bridge and a cosmic telephone. I would liken it to a cosmic phone with a cosmic fax machine attached. The cosmic phone rep-

9. Distance Healing

resents being able to connect with anyone or anything in the universe. The cosmic fax machine (or bridge) means you can send the healing energy of Reiki and the Reiki symbols, as well as affirmations, positive words and intentions to the person or people you connect with. Therefore the Distance symbol has two functions during distance healing. The first is to connect and the second is to provide the means by which Reiki and the symbols can be sent across time and distance.

Because Reiki is healing energy it cannot be used for negative intentions. It always moves towards a healing. The promises of the Twelve Yaksha Generals and the Guardians of Healing (Sunlight and Moonlight) also stipulate that whenever the Healing Buddha's name is used people will be protected from evil. The Healing Buddha's name is used in the Distance symbol as the Character Ki (Wood).

If it is not in the best interest of Receivers to receive Reiki they will not get it no matter how many people send them Distance Healing. If people block receiving Reiki they will also not get it. However, once the blocks are cleared any Reiki that has been sent to them, either in the past or present, will begin working in their lives. This also applies to people receiving a hands-on Reiki treatment or a Reiki initiation. Therefore it can be said that one of the natural laws of Reiki is that it is the receiver who decides how much energy they get and whether they will accept it or not. The intentions, affirmations and positive words sent during Distance Healing will only work if they are in the best interest of the person receiving the healing. Distance Healing always works for the highest good of the person receiving it, not for the person sending it. On one occasion a student of mine rang me to ask why, as she had sent her husband lots and lots of Reiki, he still wasn't obeying her? Reiki just does not work that way. Distance Healing is not only about healing but also about honouring the Buddha within the person you are sending to.

Reiki helps us to travel through each day, each week, each year of our lives easily, safely and happily. Reiki will only work for us in our lives if we use it. This can be done by giving ourselves regular self-treatments and by using the Reiki symbols for anything that we find difficult, upsetting, boring and tiring. Working daily with the Reiki symbols will bring more energy, excitment and interest into our lives.

Chapter 10

THE SPIRITUAL LINEAGE BEARER
MASTER SYMBOL - 4th Symbol of Reiki

The Reiki Master symbol is the spiritual lineage bearer of Reiki. This symbol enables Reiki and its attunement/initiation system to be passed from Master to student. It is the vital ingredient which ensures Reiki attunements/initiations actually work. The Reiki Master symbol is traditionally taught at 3rd Degree Reiki, which is also the spiritual level of Reiki.

Origin

The Reiki Master symbol can be seen as a vase/jar on the foot of the Healing Buddha at Yakushi-ji in Nara, Japan. It symbolises our wholeness—all that we are made of (clay—physical level); all that we contain (space within—mental/emotional level); all that makes us who we are (a container of all of life's experiences, in balance and oneness—spiritual level); and all that we can become (the leaves coming out of the vase—cosmic level). In *Sky Dancer*, Keith Dowman likens the vase to the chalice or Holy Grail in the legends of King Arthur.

The Japanese version (as found in a English/Japanese dictionary) of the Reiki Master symbol contains 17 strokes, the same as the number of spokes in the central wheel on the foot of Yakushi (the Healing Buddha) which represents the journey of Reiki and the energetic pattern of the healing energy of the universe. The name of the Reiki Master symbol is the same as the name for the 34th Past Buddha. Consequently I believe that the number 17 is the vibrational number of Reiki, with 34 being its master number and 51, the number of Buddhas and Bodhisattvas in the Healing Buddha mandala, being the cosmic number of Reiki.

The foremost importance of the Reiki Master symbol is its use in Reiki initiations/attunements. Because a symbol has many functions it can also be used in other areas of your life; for your spiritual journey and to manifest form or energy.

Interpretation of the Symbol

The Reiki Master symbol was most likely developed in China where the sutras of the Healing Buddha were fully evolved. Only one version of the Healing Buddha sutras has been found in India, at Gilgit, and it is very brief. In the Reiki story Mrs Takata says that Mikao Usui learned Chinese so that he could study the sutras in that language.

I believe that the first two vows made by the Healing Buddha describes the construction of the bija symbol, or symbol for the subtle body, of the Healing Buddha. The Reiki Master Symbol fits the description of the bija symbol for the Healing Buddha. The most comprehensive English translation of the Healing Buddha's vows appear in the book *The Healing Buddha* by Raoul Birnbaum.

Dai means Great. The horizontal stroke represents the number one and the other two strokes represents man (as in human). A No 1 Man was a "great man" therefore this symbol came to mean "Great". Buddhists also interpret this symbol as: Mysterious; Excellent; and All Powerful. In the description of the first vow made by the Healing Buddha it states that the body of the Healing Buddha will have the marks of a great man. The Dai, therefore, represents the marks of a

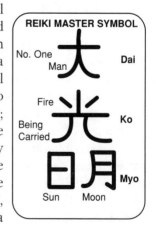

great man. The "great man" is, I believe,comparable with the "superior man" described in the *I Ching*.

10. THE SPIRITUAL LINEAGE BEARER

Ko means light. In the past a light was fire carried on a stick, and so this character is based on "fire being carried. The top three strokes represent fire. The lower three strokes represent "being carried by man" with the last two strokes being a pair of legs moving. Hence the original meaning of this symbol was "Fire being carried by man." In the Healing Buddha's first vow it states that a light will blaze from his body and that sentient beings will be able to have a body like the Healing Buddha's body. Both of these concepts can be found depicted within the character of Ko which can mean "Man carrying a light that blazes (ie fire)". Later, as the use of light became more sophisticated, the Ko character was used to mean a lamp and now it refers to any light. In the past the Healing Buddha monks would light big lamps when doing healing work.

Myo which is the sun and moon characters shown together, means bright or brightness. The sun and the moon together symbolises a light brighter than either one on its own and therefore can mean brightness and also clarity. The second vow of the Healing Buddha mentions that the subtle body of the Healing Buddha will have a radiance brighter than the sun and moon. These two characters can also be interpreted as day and night. Buddhists use this symbol to mean: To be clear; Universal wisdom; Knowledge and learning.

The Reiki Master symbol can be interpreted as *"Great Light of Brightness"* or *"Great Light of the Sun and Moon"*. Yet another way of looking at this symbol is: *"A great man carries the Light day and night"*. It can also be translated as *"Big (Dai) Enlightenment (Ko Myo)"*.

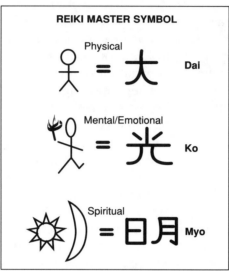

According to ancient western Mysteries Schools, man made in the image of God, has three parts—spirit, body and soul. The spirit was seen as male, the body as earthy and therefore female and it was said that when the spirit and body came together in union they created the soul. The Greek Mysteries described the soul as "a radiant body of light", calling it "augoeides" which means "form of radiance". Although Buddhists do not believe in a soul, they also describe man as having three parts—body, mind and spirit. The Reiki Master symbol appears to support the idea that when body and mind come together they create the spirit as a light brighter than the sun and moon.

Like the Distance symbol, other characters can be found within the Reiki Master symbol—symbols for cosmic beings; symbols for initiation; and a trinity (Heaven/Human/Earth) which enables you to remain balanced during your journey, during the initiation, and during your interaction with higher beings or energies.

10. THE SPIRITUAL LINEAGE BEARER

Cosmology of the Symbol

At 1st and 2nd Degree levels of Reiki I was led to believe that doing Reiki involved just channelling energy from somewhere in the universe. At 3rd Degree level I was introduced to the idea that we work with Higher Beings, who exist on another plane, similar to or the same as Angels. During my Reiki Master training I was told to decide on what Higher Beings I would like to work with during the initiations. Being a very practical, feet on the ground, type of person I found this idea very hard to accept. I was not sure about being a Reiki Master if I had take on such a concept. I finally decided I could accept working with my Spiritual Guide and Ascended Reiki Masters but didn't really believe I would actually have their assistance during an initiation.

Early Reiki initiations that I gave to students amazed me. My students reported seeing visions of two Buddhist monks in yellow robes assisting me and feeling their hands on them during the initiations. They also saw people in the room with us who looked like Egyptians (perhaps they were Babylonians or Assyrians), and Hindu Indians. I've never seen anyone myself but often I feel a presence assisting me and sometimes experience my face transfiguring so that it feels as though I am wearing a pair of glasses perched on my nose–sometimes the name Mikao Usui whispers through my mind and at other times it's Chujiro Hayashi's name. Gradually I have come to accept such phenomena during an initiation and welcome such Beings who assist me. At no time have I or any of my students been harmed by such experiences. I believe that Reiki protects us throughout the initiation and the class.

The Reiki Master symbol encompasses bijas for higher energies/beings who assist in the initiation process. Overall this symbol is the subtle body of a great Enlightened Being (Buddha) which when activated in a healing initiation becomes the subtle body of the Healing Buddha. At the same time it contains within it the subtle bodies (symbols) of other energies or beings. Although Japanese would not read the Reiki Master symbol in this way, I have found that it helps me to understand the symbol better.

Dai

In Japanese Buddhism the character of Dai is used for its "blessing power" because it converts to the "power of Absolute Nature". This character is considered to be "All powerful".

These characters, which can mean "Light of the Sun and Moon" form the name of the 34th Past Buddha. Apart from the information about the Past

Ko Myo

Buddhas as a group which appears in *Healing Buddha* and *Literary Evidence for Early Buddhist Art in China* I was unable to find anything specifically about the 34th Past Buddha. The Buddha of Sun and Moon Light is mentioned in the Lotus Sutra which was read in conjunction with the Healing Buddha sutra. The Past Buddhas are acknowledged as powerful entities who "awaken and enlighten". This Past Buddha probably has a particular affinity to the Healing Buddha's Guardian Bodhisattvas; Sunlight and Moonlight.

Dainichi

Dainichi (Vairocana) is the Buddha who personifies the central source of power in the universe. Dainichi also represents the "Great Sun" or "Light of God" which resides within each person. He is also used to represent an enlightened or illuminated mind.

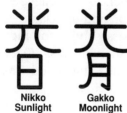

Nikko
Sunlight

Gakko
Moonlight

Sunlight and Moonlight represent the two Bodhisattvas who are the Guardians of the Healing Buddha's correct Law. They ensure that both the user and receiver are always protected when doing Reiki and when using the Reiki Master symbol.

130

10. The Spiritual Lineage Bearer

For Initiation

The Reiki Master symbol is used during the initiation process to awaken and enlighten; to illuminate the mind; to bless, protect, and convert to the healing power of the universe.

Dai (Great) Tunes into the energy, blesses and converts to the energy.

Dainichi (Great Sun) Brings in the energy from the central, creative force of the universe and illuminates the mind.

Ko Myo (Light of the Sun & Moon) Awakens and enlightens the receiver to the energy.

Nikko (Sunlight) & Gakko (Moonlight) Determines that the energy is Healing energy. Also protects Master and student during the initiation.

Myo Keeps negative/positive in balance and harmony throughout the initiation.

Integration of a Journey

Many people often find themselves going through the same experiences again and again without knowing why. They do not recognise the lessons, do not review them nor are they honest about why the experiences happen. The Reiki Master symbol assists with the processing which needs to take place at the end of a journey or experience. The journey is only successful if travellers are able to clearly understand the benefits, lessons, and knowledge experienced and are able to integrate those experiences within themselves so that they become a part of themselves. If the journey is not successful then it will need to be experienced again. The Reiki Master symbol enables this processing and integration to take place easily, and almost unconsciously. It allows the person to get off the treadmill of continuously repeating an experience. It brings light to the process. It also helps us to realise our true inner light and allows us to let our inner light, passions and talents shine for others to see. The symbol also enables us to respond automatically, rightly and wisely to similar lessons and experiences we may meet in the future and to access our inner creativity easily. It brings us greater self-awareness—but only if we use the symbol on ourselves.

People who are initiated to the Reiki Master symbol experience a sense of peace and well-being when they use this symbol. They find that many of their experiences reach a point of completion. Often they will finish off things in their lives—this may manifest as spring-cleaning or renovating their home; the completion of a cardigan they have been knitting for a year or more; or other projects which have dragged on for a long period of time; or the ending of long unhappy relationships—creating time and space for new relationships and new opportunities.

Torch in Daylight

This symbol indicates that the journey to the soul or spirit level has been reached and the knowledge and experience we gained throughout the journey has been integrated right to soul level and can now be reflected back out to the rest of the world as a shining light. It signifies that the journey continues at a higher level, with greater light, clarity and strength. For to carry a light as bright as the sun requires strength. The strength to know what is right and wrong, what is positive and negative, to maintain peace and harmony and a strong sense of equilibrium. Always being able to stay in balance maintains strength. The things we have integrated to the depths of our soul are the seeds which will grow and nourish us.

Mikao Usui stood in the market place holding a "Torch in Daylight".

10. The Spiritual Lineage Bearer

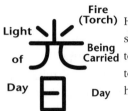

Torch in Daylight

He became a "shining example of Reiki", able to shine the light from within out to the world. Able to withstand the negative comments of others and to maintain a positive, joyful attitude towards both himself and others.

Using the Reiki Master symbol

Within the 12 vows of the Healing Buddha can be found some of the things that the Reiki Master symbol can used for. In summary these are to:

Never lack the necessities of life.

Remain on the path of enlightenment.

Follow the rules of conduct perfectly, commit no faults, act in a wholesome manner and benefit all sentient beings.

Improve their sense organs and not suffer or be sick.

Be peaceful and joyous in body and mind and have plentiful families and property.

Transform a negative way of life to a positive attitude to life.

Gradually cultivate and study the practices of a spiritual journey.

Be free from all sorrows and sufferings caused by the King's laws.

Be provided with food and drink to satisfy their bodies.

Be able to obtain clothing, precious adornment, incense, music and other arts.

The Vows of the Healing Buddha are symbolic and can be difficult to understand and seem to be very old-fashioned and out-dated. The vow which I have summarised as *"Be free from all sorrows and sufferings caused by the King's laws"* can be referred back to the spiritual journey where the "King" represents the highest authority who sets the laws and rules that you live by. Many of us carry around a lot of instructions and rules set by our families which can cause us to be very unhappy. The Master symbol can therefore free us from the injunctions and belief patterns we carry about as excess baggage which hold us down or hold us back or which we

133

struggle with throughout our lives.

The vow which I have referred to as *"Provided with food and drink to satisfy their bodies"* can mean that we will gradually change our tastes in food and drink until what we eat and drink is more beneficial for our bodies. At the same time many of us eat because we are dissatisfied with the life we are living. Reiki and the Reiki Master symbol will help provide us with the interests and stimulation which will enable us to enjoy living our lives in a satisfying way. Clothing and precious adornment can be re-read as confidence/self-worth and the glow of good health.

Like the other Reiki symbols the Reiki Master symbol needs to be used and experienced regularly to be effective. The idea is to work with it until you become "one" with it so that its benefits operate automatically in your life daily.

Insights from Drawing the Master Symbol

Like the Power symbol and the Mental/Emotional symbol the Reiki Master symbol can show you something about yourself. Because I don't teach any other form of the Reiki Master

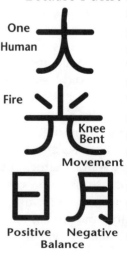

symbol I have no comment about how people draw the Dai character. As this character represents a great man it would follow that those who do not draw it correctly will have trouble with "greatness" which may explain why some Reiki Masters have trouble rising above pettiness, competitiveness and one-up-manship. I have noticed that those people who rush through the Reiki system tend to draw the Master symbol so that the fire is jammed up against the character for human; as though their "bums are on fire". If there is a large gap between the Dai and the Ko then they are slow learners, who get there in the end.

When both the legs of the Ko are drawn exactly the same the person tends to come to a stand still after becoming a Master. The two different strokes represent the legs moving—when you walk or run one knee will bend as the other straightens. They seem to indicate movement along the spiritual pathway.

If the sun character is drawn with gaps in the outside strokes it indicates a person who appears to speak positively but is actually talking about negative things like road accidents, murders, how badly someone does something, etc; allowing their positive attitude to leak away. If the sun character is bigger than the moon character then the person tends to be overly enthusiastic, positive, left-brained and is out of balance. If the moon character is out of proportion to the sun then these people tend to put themselves down and regularly apologise for things they say and do; or are very introspective.

Many people draw their sun and moon symbols with a Z inside them. These people have simply recorded the hand movement from the inside stroke to the final closing stroke of the symbol. It may indicate that these people are very much connected with outside appearances and what other people think of them.

The Non-Traditional Master Symbol

Some Reiki lineages have chosen not to teach the Reiki Master symbol, rejecting it as the "Traditional" Master symbol preferring to use the symbol often known as the Tibetan or Non-traditional Master symbol. The Reiki Master symbol is an integral component of the Usui System of Reiki. To leave it out of your Reiki training is to lose a very valuable and important aspect of Reiki. Such a pity. The Tibetan or Non-traditional Master symbol, which uses a fire symbol from the fire (Amitabha) mandala, has been given the same name as the Reiki Master symbol. During Reiki initiations only the name of the symbol will be working as a fire symbol has little or no relevancy to a Reiki initiation which belongs to a water (Healing Buddha) mandala. The Reiki Master symbol protects, balances and brings in the correct energies to a Reiki initiation. It allows for the full integration of Reiki and the Reiki experience. It has no substitute or equivalent, that I know of, which can do all that.

Chapter 11

REIKI INITIATIONS

I have chosen not to describe a Reiki initiation in this book. Each lineage appears to have a different format for doing an initiation and as each works, I cannot say which format is the correct one. However, I would like to share the following insights:

Controlling the Energy Flow

In the past it was believed that the Reiki Master could control how much energy passed from master to student. Consequently Reiki Masters have done such things as hold their breath during the entire initiation, often causing hyperventilation after three or four initiations; or hold their tongues to the roof of their mouths while holding the Hui Yin point. My experience has led me to believe that it is not the Reiki Master who determines how strong the energy will be during an initiation but rather the student who decides the amount of energy they receive in just the same way that it is the receiver who decides how much energy they accept during a Reiki treatment or when receiving Distance Healing. Therefore it is recommended that the receiver be as relaxed as possible and that they have a trust in the person doing the initiation.

Blocks

If there is a lack of trust for any reason the receiver can partially or wholly block the initiation. If at any time a Reiki Master believes that someone has unconsciously blocked an initiation because of an old inhibition they can use the Power symbol to clear away the block either during the initiation process or after it during a Reiki treatment. Although the energy may have been blocked it is still there waiting for the receiver to access it at any time without needing to go through a further initiation. However, if an initiation has been consciously blocked the Reiki Master may not be able to clear the block—the blockage needs to be cleared by the person receiving the initiation.

The block may be because the receiver has placed "white light" around themselves just before the initiation, showing that they do not fully trust Reiki or the Reiki Master. Another reason may be due to the Reiki Master not fully explaining Reiki leaving the receiver worried about whether they are doing the right thing or not. On one occasion I had a student who believed she was not able to receive very much life force energy because she had been sickly most of her life. After her initiation she had no energy at all coming through her hands. I gave her a Reiki treatment which began with my using the Power symbol and an intent to clear her belief that she could not receive the life force energy. Shortly after the treatment started the young Japanese woman happily announced that the energy was flowing through her hands very strongly. Young adults pushed to Reiki classes by their enthusiastic parents may also have a resistance to Reiki initiations.

If you believe that you may have blocked your Reiki initiations at 1st, 2nd or 3rd Degree levels it is possible to clear away the blocks and allow the effects of the initiations to work more strongly in your life. It is advisable to do this at the beginning of a full self-treatment by placing your hands on yourself and stating three times that you are now willing to let go of the beliefs you held at the time of your Reiki initiations that prevented you from being strongly and clearly connected with Reiki. Then use the Power symbol.

11. Reiki Initiations

Attunement or Initiation

Using the word "initiation" during the preparation period of a Reiki initiation/attunement when you set your intent instead of the word "attunement" appears to be more powerful. Probably because the word "initiation" is older and has been used for such rituals far longer. An initiation encompasses the whole experience of Reiki—unfolding as the initiate learns through processing each lesson presented by their relationships, experiences and environment. An attunement simply means access to the energy.

Channel for Reiki

The Reiki Master acts as a channel or conduit for the energy during the initiation. They are not the origin of the energy nor do they own it. The format of the initiation is symbolic and acts as a directive which provokes a response from the Universal Life Force Energy. Some of the symbols used in the initiation process are:

Grabbing the Thunderbolt—in *The Healing Buddha* by Raoul Birnbaum the Lama is said to visualise himself seizing the thunderbolt in both hands before an initiation. I believe this is the equivalent to a Reiki Master drawing the Power symbol (thunderbolt) on both palms before they begin an initiation. The metaphor of "seizing the thunderbolt" seems to indicate that drawing the Power symbol should not be done in a wish-washy way but with vigour and concentration.

Stepping into the Mandala—Healing Buddha initiations are performed within a Healing Buddha mandala. The Lama does this by visualising himself entering the mandala. I believe Reiki Masters do this when they Reiki the room where they do initiations and hold their classes by drawing the Power symbol at all the directions, north, south, east, west, SE, SW, NE and NW and on the ceiling and floor. This acts as a protecting field—similar to the vajras which surround the mandala and also acknowledges the Kings and Guardians of the Directions. A Lama faces east when doing initiations. This is the direction the Buddha was facing when he reached "enlightenment". It was also the direction Mikao Usui faced when sitting on top of the mountain—"*he saw a light coming straight at him from the east*".

Merging with the Healing Buddha—Some Lamas spiritually merge with the vibrations of the Healing Buddha before entering the mandala and some do so after they enter it. As the Reiki Master Symbol is the subtle or vibrational body of the Healing Buddha this simply means merging with the Reiki Master symbol. This can be done by drawing a large symbol (same size as yourself) and stepping into it as you say its name.

Birth of a Buddha—My lineage does not teach the Reiki Master to hold one hand above their head while doing an initiation and for a long time I could not understand why such a hand position was necessary until I saw a picture of a statue of a Buddha pointing his right hand towards the sky and his left hand towards the earth. This hand position represents the birth of a Buddha—the birth of the Buddha Within who stands between above (Heaven) and below (Earth). Therefore this hand mudra, I believe, can be used in a Reiki initiation to awaken the Buddha (God) Within the initiate. I use it at the beginning of an initiation prior to placing my hands on the student.

Namesté—This has been translated as "I greet the God Within". This recognises that the Buddha/God/Christ Within has been activated by the initiation. This greeting is addressed to the student at the completion of the initiation.

Tongue on Roof of Mouth—In some Reiki lineages Masters rest the tips of their tongues on the roof of their mouths throughout the initiation. This is supposed to provide a channel for the energy to flow down the front of the Master's body. According to Pobangka Rinpoche in *Liberation in the Palm of Your Hand,* placing the tongue on your palate ensures your mouth does not dry out and it also prevents saliva from running out of your mouth.

Blowing—During an initiation Reiki Masters blow their breath down the front of the initiate. This symbolises the Universal Life Force Energy entering the initiate. During Tibetan Buddhist initiations the Master begins blowing at the left nostril and continues down to the base of the body then back upwards to the right nostril symbolically representing the flow of the life force energy through the nadirs—the energy lines which are said to spiral around the spine and which start and finish at the nostrils.

Crossing the Initiate's Arms—When I have finished blowing on the initiate I cross their arms so their hands are resting on the front of their shoulders. Several people asked me why and my reply had always been: "this was the way I was taught." Later I discovered that this hand position in Buddhism means "Victory over Ignorance, Hate and Violence".

Holding Your Arms Out when Blessing the Initiate— this symbolises the "Dai" of the Reiki Master symbol. The Master should stand with feet apart and arms held horizontally, head up and body in balance. The "Dai" bestows a blessing from the universe. You can also intend that your initiate always remains in balance and harmony. When done properly it can feel very balancing, beautiful and sacred.

Healing Buddha Mudra—I have chosen to complete my initiations with the Healing Buddha Mudra. I do this after the Dai Blessing and before bringing my palms together and saying Namesté. The left hand is: arm held straight down, fingertips pointing to the ground and palm facing the initiate. This signifies a blessing from the Great Mother. The right hand is: arm straight up, fingertips pointing toward heaven, and the thumb and middle finger bent forward but not touching, palm facing the initiate. This signifies courage bestowed from Heaven, a gift to the initiate about to embark on the journey of the mandala, which will assist them through the journey.

Four Initiations at 1st Degree Reiki

Although I was taught to give one initiation to a 1st Degree Reiki student, and I know that one is all that is necessary to connect the student to Reiki, my search has brought me to the realisation that the ideal number of initiations for 1st Degree Reiki is four. The 1st Degree Reiki initiations not only activate the flow of the Universal Life Force Energy they also open the gateways to the four levels—1st initiation = physical level (East gate), 2nd initiation = mental/emotional level (South gate), 3rd initiation = spiritual level (West gate), and 4th initiation = cosmic level (North gate). It allows Reiki to flow to each of these levels easily and quickly without it being blocked. In the Reiki story it says Mikao Usui sat at the top of the mountain for 21 days. I believe "top of the mountain" can be interpreted as reaching the cosmic level by moving through all four levels.

Because changes have come about in the practice of Reiki since Mrs Takata died, not all Reiki Masters give four initiations during a 1st Degree Reiki class. At first glance it would seem incorrect not to open all gates of the energy in a student. However, its seems to me that although anyone can be initiated to Reiki not all students are able, or allowed, to have all four of their gates open. Having Reiki Masters who only open one gate has made Reiki available to more people—people who want Reiki in only one part of their lives, not in all areas of it.

In Hinduism the four cardinal points of east, south, west and north were considered to be lands or continents ruled by Kings known as Wheel (chakra) Kings. The wheel was a sign of dominion or rulership and a Chakra or Wheel King was able to travel all over his land or continent; the more wheels he had the more lands or directions he could travel. When the King gained dominionship of his land or lands he became known as a Universal Monach. In *The Buddhist Praying Wheel* William Simpson describes the Universal Monarchs as:

The golden-wheel King	-righteously rules all four directions or continents
The silver-wheel King	-rules three directions
The copper-wheel King	-rules two directions
The iron-wheel King	-rules one direction

A Universal Monach who, like the Buddha at the centre of a mandala, rules from the centre of the four wheels of east, south, west and north was known as a "Holy" King who could traverse the universe according to his thoughts.

These various kings are an acknowledgement of people who have complete control or rulership of one area of their lives but not another—for instance the business whiz who is so competent, efficient and successful at work, but unhappy and unsuccessful in marriage and family life at home.

In Buddhism the Chakra Kings are affiliated to the Five Dhyani Buddhas.

Aksobhya	**East**	**Blue**	**Heart Chakra**
Ratnasambhava	**South**	**Yellow**	**Solar Plexus**
Amitabha	**West**	**Red**	**Throat Chakra**
Amoghasiddhi	**North**	**Green**	**Sacral Chakra**
Vairocana	**Centre**	**White**	**Brow Chakra**

Sealing the Initiation

Traditionally, the first three initiations of 1st Degree are unsealed and the fourth one is sealed. In Buddhism the seal is used to "not go beyond". An initiation is unsealed when there is to be another initiation to follow and sealed when there are no more initiations beyond it. For instance the initiation which activates the ability to use Reiki on the cosmic level is sealed because there is nothing beyond the cosmic level, but the other three levels are unsealed because there is always another level beyond each of them. The initiations for the symbols are also sealed because the Reiki symbols are in the spiritual form of the symbols and as there are no symbols in the cosmic level there are no higher forms of the Reiki symbols.

1st initiation	Physical level of Reiki	unsealed
2nd initiation	Mental/emotional level of Reiki	unsealed
3rd initiation	Spiritual level of Reiki	unsealed
4th initiation	Cosmic level of Reiki	sealed
5th initiation	Activating the 2nd Degree symbols	sealed
6th initiation	Activating the Master symbol	sealed

One Initiation at 2nd Degree Reiki

I have heard it said that to attune a practitioner to three symbols in one initiation has a scrambling effect. To me there appears to be little foundation for this belief. David Neil in *Tibetan Buddhism* records an initiation where three symbols are placed in the hands during an initiation while Michael Saso in *Tantric Art and Meditation* describes an initiation for just one symbol. It seems that the number of symbols activated during an initiation is a matter of choice by the initiating Reiki Master.

The Tibetan initiation, which placed three symbols in the hands, puts the Vajra (Power Symbol) in the right hand, the Ah (Mental/Emotional Symbol) in the left hand, and the wheel (not used in Reiki) in both hands. This seems to indicate the symbols for 2nd Degree Reiki could be activated in the hands as the Power Symbol in the right hand (Positive-Yang Energy), the Mental/Emotional Symbol in the left hand (Negative-Yin Energy) and the Distance Symbol drawn over both hands at once, to balance positive and negative (Neutral-Yin/Yang Energy). However, my preference would be to put each of the symbols in both hands—once over the right hand, once over the left hand and then over both hands together, because the Sanskrit word "pani" is plural and therefore means both hands.

Chapter 12

THE REIKI STORY—ITS ESOTERIC MEANINGS

One day my son asked me if I believed the Reiki Story and how Mikao Usui rediscovered Reiki. After listening to me tell the story during a Reiki class he told me that I related the story as though I didn't believe it. His question made me realise that I didn't really know what to believe about the Reiki Story yet deep in my heart I knew that the Reiki Story was an important aspect of Reiki; I just didn't know why.

As a descendant of William Rand's Reiki lineage I was aware that there was no record of Mikao Usui attending Chicago University and nor had he ever been the head of a Christian School in Japan. It was believed that Mrs Takata had added the Christian aspect to the Reiki Story so Reiki would be more appealing to Christians in the USA. For me, because this part of the Story was not true, it jeopardised the credibility of the rest of Mikao Usui's story. I kept teaching the Reiki Story during 1st Degree classes while looking for a way of understanding the story so that it would have a credible meaning for myself and my students.

According to several sources, Mikao Usui was born in Japan in the Gifu District on 15 August 1865 and died in Fukuyama, Hiroshima on 9 March 1926. Toshitaka Mochizuki, author of *Iyashi No Te*, believes that although Mikao Usui probably had a Buddhist education he was neither a Christian nor a Buddhist monk. The inscription on Mikao Usui's memorial stone does confirm that he discovered Reiki and was the founder of Usui method of Reiki, but it does not tell the Reiki story the way we in the west know it.

As I searched through books about Buddhism for a greater understanding of Reiki I began to realise that the Buddhist stories and sutras were written for more than one level of understanding. On the first level a story is simply an entertaining anecdote for anyone to hear. However, on a second level the story has a psychological meaning and acts as a guide to coping with certain aspects of living. On a third level it has a deeper, metaphysical meaning. I looked at the Reiki Story from this point of view and found that it could indeed be viewed from all three levels. Discovering that "Torch in Daylight" can be found both within the Reiki Master symbol and the Reiki story confirmed for me that not only was it an entertaining story, and a psychological story, but that it also contained a metaphysical message.

In Buddhism unveiling the deeper messages of a story often takes many years and each person comes to their "enlightenment" of the story in their own time and way through meditation as well as reading, writing and reciting the story thousands of times. For Mikao Usui's original students this aspect of story-telling would have been familiar. However, in the west students are unfamiliar with looking for deeper meanings and hidden metaphysical knowledge within a story that on the surface appears to be someone's personal history, although we are familiar with myths and fairy tales which are similar kinds of stories.

Mircea Elaide suggests that myths and fairy tales are psychodramatic expressions of initiation rites associated with transformation to higher planes of existence. The difference between a myth and a fairy tale is said to be in the ending of the story—a myth nearly always ends tragically, while fairy tales have happy endings. Fairy tales use the language of symbols to appeal to both our conscious and subconscious minds simultaneously. They suggest answers depending on what questions the initiate asks and on what difficulties they are having in finding their higher self. Therefore a fairy tale can have a variety of interpretations.

In my opinion the Reiki Story is a very skilfully composed metaphysical fairy tale which externalises the inner journey that Reiki takes its initiates on. I believe that the addition of the much disputed Christian segment to the Reiki story was skilfully done, not just to make it easier to teach Reiki to Christians but to act as a Rosetta stone to enable Christians to interpret the Reiki Story.

The Reiki Story

It has been said that Mikao Usui, who rediscovered Reiki, was the principal of a Christian school near Kyoto. One day he was challenged by his students to show them how to heal with his hands, the way Jesus did. Unable to do so, Mikao Usui is said to have given up his position as principal and travelled to the USA to study theology at Chicago University. After seven years of study, and failing to discover how to heal with his hands, Mikao Usui returned home to Japan.

In Japan Mikao Usui continued his search by travelling from monastery to monastery asking if anyone knew how to heal with their hands. He was told that "We did know once, but don't know now. We now heal only the mind, not the body." Finally Mikao Usui came to a Zen Monastery in Kyoto where he was invited to stay and study. The Abbot believed that if someone was truly dedicated and does not give up they would achieve their quest. The Abbot also believed that if something was known once, it could be known again.

It has been said that Mikao Usui stayed at the monastery for many years studying the sacred writings of Buddhism. He learned Chinese and Sanskrit so he could also study the sutras in those languages. It was while studying the Buddhist sutras that he found a formula for contacting a higher being who could bestow the gift of healing. After discussion with the Abbot, Mikao Usui went to a sacred mountain outside Kyoto where he intended to fast, meditate and chant as described in the formula he found. He asked the Abbot to send out a search party for him if he did not return within 22 days.

Mikao Usui set 21 stones before him and threw one away each day to keep track of time. On the last day, just before dawn, Mikao Usui saw a bright, shining light coming towards him from the east at great speed. Realising that if he avoided the light he would not discover what he was searching for Mikao Usui stayed where he was and allowed the light to hit him. As the beam of light hit him on his forehead (third eye) he was knocked over, unconscious. He then saw hundreds of coloured bubbles which contained symbols and information about Reiki. Around midday Mikao Usui regained consciousness. He felt refreshed and energised. He hurried down the mountain to tell the Abbot what had happened.

On his way down the mountain Mikao Usui stubbed his toe. Sitting down he automatically held his toe between his hands. To his surprise the pain stopped and when he looked the injury had healed. At the bottom of the mountain he stopped at a wayside Inn where he met the innkeeper's granddaughter who had a toothache. Mikao Usui asked if he could place his hands on the young lady's face. When he did so the swelling went down and the aching went away. Mikao Usui then asked for a meal. The innkeeper warned that the meal Mikao Usui ordered was too large for someone who had been fasting. Mikao ate the meal without any ill effects.

On his return to the Zen monastery Mikao Usui bathed, changed his clothes, and requested an audience with the

12. THE REIKI STORY—ITS ESOTERIC MEANINGS

Abbot. While they discussed how he could use his gift of heal-ing, Mikao Usui healed the old Abbot's arthritis. Eventually it was decided that Mikao would go to the Beggar City in Kyoto so he could help the poor and destitute to have better lives. It is said he worked there for seven years.

Mikao Usui chose to heal the young men in the Beggar City. They, he believed, healed quicker than the old because they had less mental/emotional problems attached to their ill health. Once he had given them Reiki he sent the young men to the monastery for a new set of clothes, a new name and a job. One day Mikao Usui realised that he was seeing the same young men again. He asked why they had returned to the Beggar City. Their reply was that it was easier to beg and steal than to change their lives and work for a living. Deeply upset, some say he fell down with his face in the mud. It was then that Mikao Usui realised that he was healing the body but not the spirit or the mind.

Returning to the monastery Mikao Usui spent time med-itating on Reiki and how to use Reiki so that the healing was permanent. After a period of meditation Mikao Usui decid-ed that adding the Five Principles to the Reiki would make it more effective. Mikao Usui also came to the conclusion that there needed to be an energy exchange so the gift of Reiki would be appreciated. He also decided that he would not push Reiki on anyone and everyone, but to pass it on to those people who were interested and wanted Reiki in their lives.

Mikao Usui then began travelling around Japan, from village to village and town to town teaching Reiki. In broad daylight he would stand on a street corner or in the local marketplace with a large lighted torch. People would laugh at him and point out to him that it was already daylight, and there was no need to carry a lighted torch. Usui would reply that if they were interested he could teach them how *to have more light, enjoyment and health in their lives. Mikao Usui would then invite them to go to a nearby temple, either in the afternoon or evening, to listen to him talk about Reiki. He would wait at the temple and teach Reiki to those who were interested enough to come along to listen to him.*

The Reiki Story is not really the personal history of Mikao Usui. It is about the journey each one of us undertakes when we become initiated to Reiki.

The Christian Version

Applying Taoist and Buddhist interpretations to the Reiki story of the journey of discovery made by Mikao Usui gives it a profound significance. The ages of people can indicate their place on a mandala or their role in a story. The young men who challenged Mikao Usui's faith in Christianity indicate that Usui's reason for starting his journey of discovery came from the wrong direction and would ultimately fail, which is indeed what happened. Usui did not find Reiki within the Christian teachings. The young men in the Beggar City indicate that Mikao Usui's experience there would likewise end in failure, which it did. He had to return to the monastery to do further meditation and study. A spiritual journey should begin with a strong desire which comes from within ourselves but which blossoms when we receive guidance from a parental type figure. In many ancient stories, fairy tales and legends about a heroic or spiritual journey, the hero is given help or advice by a wise old man or woman. This happens when Mikao Usui meets the Abbot of the Monastery in Kyoto.

On a metaphysical level the Christian story represents a false start to Mikao Usui's search for Reiki. This part of the Reiki Story tells us that the spiritual search or journey does not require us to travel to a far distant place. Mikao Usui's return home to Japan indicates that our spiritual journey starts from home, the place we are familiar with. In ancient times the hearth of a home was held sacred as both the centre of the home and the place from which a journey began and to which the traveller returned. Home can also mean that part within us which is our true self or inner spirit or essence. Also when setting out to discover something you will travel a long way from where you started; ie: from the place of ignorance to a state of knowledge. Once you have learned all you can that information and experience will find a home within yourself so that it becomes a part of you, your talents and knowledge.

The Christian segment appears to give us some definitions. The word "Japan" means home and home can mean our body which is the home of our soul/self or Buddha/Christ. The words Christianity and USA can be defined respectively as a philosophy or belief system, and a the place where a philosophy is studied ie: Mikao Usui studied Christian theology in the USA. This indicates to me that Mikao Usui may never have left Japan, that his travels can represent a journey around the segments of the Healing Buddha mandala which are often called Lands or countries. The first segment is related to the philosophy and theology of Buddha Sakyamuni.

There may also have been two more reasons for including Christian aspects into Reiki. During Mikao Usui's life (1865-1926) the Buddhists in Japan were involved in a battle to prevent Christianity from entering their country. The law preventing Christianity being preached or taught in Japan was not repealed until the 1870s. The mention of Christianity and Buddhism within the story tells us, I believe, that the practitioners of Reiki can rise above such squabbles between religions; Reiki can be practiced by anyone whether Christian,

Buddhist, or any other religion.

Another reason for Christianity being included may have been to indicate to Christians that the Reiki Story is similar to the stories told by Jesus: a parable! Jesus indicated that his stories contain hidden (esoteric) knowledge which is revealed when the student is ready to understand it.

The Desire to Heal with His Hands

For whatever reason, whether because he was challenged by a student or because he had experienced illness Mikao Usui developed a desire to learn how to heal with his hands. (Frank Ajarva Petter, in *Reiki Fire*, says Mikao Usui suffered from a serious illness.)

A journey always needs a goal otherwise there is no point in taking a journey. You will not stay focused nor will you know where you are going or when you have arrived. Many people in the west undertake their spiritual journey without first establishing a goal. They then drift this way and that, follow one teacher and then another and another (whoever is the latest fashion) having no sense of arrival nor fully benefiting from the gifts and insights that have been presented to them by the various courses and lectures they attend. They endlessly search because they are on a quest but never find anything because they have not set a goal. The journey is the lesson and the goal is the gift for learning the lesson. The progress towards any set goal can become a spiritual journey. In Reiki the goal is to heal yourself physically, mentally/emotionally and spiritually so you can then access the cosmic level of enlightenment.

The Search

On his return to Japan Mikao Usui continued his search by travelling from monastery to monastery around Japan asking if anyone knew how to heal with their hands.

12. THE REIKI STORY—ITS ESOTERIC MEANINGS

He was told that "We did know once, but don't know now. We now heal only the mind, not the body."

When we develop a desire to discover our life's pathway we tend to travel from idea to idea, modality to modality, often finding that they will teach us a part of what we are looking for–healing methods for the body, religion for the spirit, psychology for the mind and emotions—none of which, when taken on their own, can be called wholistic. True healing is always wholistic; healing the mind/emotions, body and spirit. A true spiritual pathway is also wholistic.

This part of the story is also a key to the meaning of the word "monastery"—the place where the mind is healed. That place is 2nd Degree Reiki. It can also signify that on the second level of the Healing Buddha mandala each of the Bodhisattva families are like separate monasteries, and all heal the mind.

The Zen Monastery

Finally Mikao Usui came to a Zen Monastery in Kyoto where he was invited to stay and study. The Abbot believed that if someone was truly dedicated and does not give up they would achieve their quest. The Abbot also believed that if something was known once, it can be known again.

This part of the story could indicate that the Zen philosophy of living in the now, detached from emotion and the results of action, is a philosophy which is compatible with Reiki. When journeying along our life's pathway it is best to remember to live in the present, day by day, rather than forever looking into the future for something better or at the past with regret. Zen is also a form of meditation which can be a tool to assist us during the journey.

Zen Buddhism also utilises esoteric meanings for words and this part of the story can act as a pointer to indicate such words are contained within the story and that Zen Buddhism can provide the interpretations of those words—in other words the Reiki Story is a koan; a puzzle which leads you to a greater awareness of your Self.

On another level the Abbot represents a spiritual mentor or guide to whom we can go for help and guidance. This mentor can often appear in our lives as a Reiki Master, a Guru, an author or some other person who has a deep understanding of life. He can also represent the spiritual level of a mandala, and also the God-self or Buddhahood contained within us.

The monastery can represent yourself, especially that still inner part of yourself which you discover during meditation. Jack Kornfield, *A Path with Heart*, says that when we sit on a meditation cushion we become our own monastery.

The Study

It has been said that Mikao Usui stayed at the monastery for many years studying the sacred writings of Buddhism. He studied them in Japanese, Chinese and Sanskrit. It was while studying the Buddhist sutras that he found a formula for contacting a higher being who could bestow the gift of healing.

Buddhism travelled from India to China and then on to Japan. About the same time that Buddhism arrived in Japan it was taken into Tibet when two princesses, one from China and one from Nepal, married the King of Tibet. The Buddhist sutras were originally written in Sanskrit, then translated into Chinese, and from Chinese into Japanese. With each translation something was missed out. For instance, the formula for contacting a higher being was apparently not translated into Japanese.

Many people are of the belief that Reiki originated in Tibet. In studying the movement of Buddhism to Japan it would seem that this is not the case. It is highly likely that

12. THE REIKI STORY—ITS ESOTERIC MEANINGS

Reiki was known to the early Buddhists of Northern India. Healing with the hands is mentioned in the Rig Veda, a sacred book of the early Hindu, and, based on the movement of religion into India, this method of healing may have been practiced in early Mesopotamia.

In *The Healing Gods of Ancient Civilizations*, the chapter on Babylonian and Assyrian gods contains a transcription from a clay tablet of a prayer asking a kindly guardian angel to help when the person placed his hands on a sick man's head at the centre of the room. The prayer also included the positions of the sun and moon in relationship to the person praying. This appeared to me to be a description of using Reiki together with knowledge of a mandala

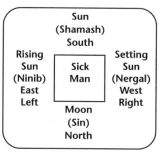

and energetic beings who assist with healing. Placing the sick man at the centre of the room may indicate he was asking for his own healing.

Kenneth Ch'en, in *Buddhism in China*, and Alexander Soper, in *Literary Evidence for Early Buddhist Art in China* both support the idea that there is a strong Persian/Iranian influence in Buddhism. Kenneth Ch'en points out that the trinity of Amitabha is similar to the trinity of the Persian deity Zurvan.

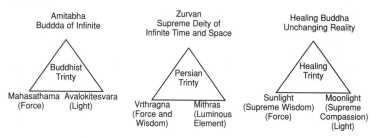

157

On another level this part of the story would indicate that the philosophies of Japan, China and India are incorporated within the philosophy of Reiki although this is not clearly apparent in the way in which Reiki is taught in the west. These philosophies are more apparent within the sutra of the Healing Buddha.

The Mountain

After discussion with the Abbot, Mikao Usui went to a sacred mountain outside Kyoto where he intended to fast, meditate and chant as described in the formula he found. He asked the Abbot to send out a search party for him if he did not return within 22 days.

The sacred mountain is Kurama which is situated outside Kyoto. The transcription of Mikao Usui's tombstone confirms that he spent 21 days at the monastery on Kurama. It should be noted that every mountain in Japan is sacred or holy.

There is an old Chinese Buddhist saying *"If you know nothing about Buddhism, mountains are mountains and waters are waters. But once you have had some instruction, mountains are no longer mountains, and waters are no longer waters."*

On a metaphysical level, in both China and Japan, a mountain represents a place of self-reflection and contemplation, a place of meditation, and does not need to be an actual mountain. This concept can be found in the *I Ching* trigram Ken which also appears in the Ba Gua map used in Feng Shui. In Buddhism the altar of a Buddha is known as a "sacred mountain". In Japan every Zen temple is considered to be a mountain and so have mountain names—even those temples situated in the middle of a city. The most amazing thing that Mikao Usui did, I believe, is to have "come down from the mountain"—in other words to have left the temple and taught Reiki to lay people so that now Reiki is available to whoever wants to learn it anywhere in the world.

Another sacred mountain can be found as a segment of a mandala. The top segment of the mountain in a mandala represents Buddhahood or oneness with the cosmic force of the universe.

The 21 Stones

Mikao Usui set 21 stones before him and threw one away each day to keep track of time.

In many societies around the world the number seven represents the completion of a spiritual journey. Twenty-one can therefore mean the completion of three journeys. The top of a mountain also symbolises achievement and the end of a journey. The twenty-one days indicates to me that Mikao Usui went through the exercises associated with the first level of the Healing Buddha's mandala and also the three journeys or pathways of the mandala.

Traditionally it is recommended that each Reiki practitioner gives themself a Reiki self-treatment each day for 21 days after being initiated to Reiki. Consciously giving yourself Reiki self-treatments for 21 days after an initiation helps to integrate the energy within your own energy field, to form a habit of giving yourself regular self-treatments and to bring about a transformation or healing within your own life.

This part of the story can also mean that each day Mikao Usui let go of old habits, beliefs and behaviours. A stone can symbolise those things that weigh you down or create obstacles and hurts in your life.

The Light

On the last day, just before dawn, Mikao Usui saw a bright shining light coming towards him at great speed.

159

Realising that if he avoided the light he would not discover what he was searching for Mikao Usui stayed where he was and allowed the light to hit him. As the beam of light hit him on his forehead (third eye) he was knocked over, unconscious. He then saw hundreds of coloured bubbles which contained symbols and information about Reiki.

This is a description of the Buddhist state of "Enlightenment". A similar description can be found in the story of Sakyamuni Buddha when he gained "enlightenment" under the Bodhi tree. In the Second Vow of the Healing Buddha it states that "he will show the dawn to beings concealed in darkness which will enable them to follow their desired paths".

It should be noted that dawn is in the east, the area where the Healing Buddha Land is said to be situated. When looking at the Healing Buddha mandala each Buddha, Bodhisattva, Yaksha and Guardian sits surrounded by a lotus petal which gives the impression of sitting inside a bubble. Each colour represents a quality—red for compassion, blue for wisdom, green for healing and yellow for insight, with white encompassing all qualities. Many Reiki people see the colour purple during a Reiki initiation. Purple, a combination of red and blue, is wisdom (Mind) and compassion (Heart) combined.

It is my belief that this experience which Mikao Usui went through is a description of the 4th Degree of Reiki; unknown within the present Reiki system. It is the step which leads to Buddhahood or total oneness with the cosmic energies of the universe. For Mikao Usui this would have meant complete oneness with the Healing Buddha (the healing energy of the universe) enabling him to become a Master of Healing. This is a very serious step. Mikao Usui was not sure he would survive the experience.

12. The Reiki Story—Its Esoteric Meanings

The Miracles

Around midday Mikao Usui regained consciousness. He felt refreshed and energised. He hurried down the mountain to tell the Abbot what had happened.

Midday can refer to the highest level of energy. Once you have completed the journey to the top of the mountain, received the enlightenment, then it is time to start the next journey up the next mountain which means starting again at the bottom of the mountain. The journey down the mountain is all about learning how to apply the enlightenment you have received. The "miracles" which are described in the Reiki story are symbols which have several meanings. They instruct us about what Reiki heals.

On his way down the mountain Mikao Usui stubbed his toe. Sitting down he automatically held his toe between his hands. To his surprise the pain stopped and when he looked the injury had healed.

This refers to the hands-on healing (physical) aspect of Reiki used to heal injuries, especially injuries which have just occurred. There are many stories in the Reiki community world-wide about injuries that have healed quickly, almost miraculously. Surgery is another type of injury to the body which responds well to Reiki treatments. The stone represents those elements which hurt us on the physical level.

At the bottom of the mountain he stopped at a wayside Inn where he met the innkeeper's granddaughter who was suffering from toothache. Mikao Usui asked if he could place his hands on the young lady's face. When he did so the swelling went down and the aching went away.

This indicates that Reiki can be used to reduce swelling and remove pain. It will remove not only physical pain but also mental and emotional pain. The girl's face, swollen with toothache, represents how we see ourselves—the face we

161

show to the world or hide from the world. The face represents our mental and emotional level. Reiki heals the pains and hurts we hold onto emotionally, and the mental attitudes which cause us pain or prevent us from moving (the girl could not afford to travel to another town to a dentist).

Placing our ten fingers (relationships) over our face during a self-treatment implies that we want our true self to be present in all our relationships, with nothing in between—no masks, no pretence, no lies or secrets, nothing that can get in the way of being ourselves with everyone we meet. Mikao Usui (man/positive) placing his hands on the young girl's face (woman/negative) signifies that the positive and negative within our relationships are brought into together in healing.

The Innkeeper's granddaughter is the only female in the story about Mikao Usui. I think she may act as a pointer to the Healing Buddha mandala which also has only one female segment in it. She represents the Great Mother or Mother Goddess within each of us who does not reveal herself until we become whole and healed. Asking for permission to place his hands on her face indicates that this part of the story is about the initiations. In Buddhism permission is sought from a Goddess before beginning an initiation.

Mikao Usui then asked for a meal. The innkeeper warned that the meal was too large for someone who had been fasting. Mikao ate the meal without any ill effects.

Reiki helps digestion and can be used to bless the food you eat. At 1st Degree Reiki you are taught to bless your food by placing your hands just above your food and giving it Reiki for a minute or so. At 2nd Degree you can bless your food by drawing the Power symbol over your food just before you eat it or while you are preparing food for a meal. Being able to Reiki their food has helped people with anorexia begin eating again. Reiki brings the vibrations of food into harmony with the body so that our mind/body and food work together to benefit us. Many Reiki practitioners gradually change their eating habits—letting go foods which are not healthy for them and learning to enjoy what they eat and to be satisfied with what they eat. On another level food represents all those things we find satisfying, stimulating and nourishing in our lives—our work, our relationships, our interests.

Eating a meal represents the spiritual level—the food represents the phsyical level; eating represents the mental/emotional level; and the energy produced by the digestion of the food represents the spiritual level. In legend the spiritual level is often represented by journeys to the Underworld. The digestion of food symbolises that journey and the transformation which comes about during it; the new energy, created by the balancing of physical and mental/emotional energies, which can be used to benefit and energise your life while enabling you to let go of all the dross/manure in your life.

The Innkeeper's warning echoes the warnings of old legends that the spiritual journey, if not done properly, or if the person is not ready, can be dangerous.

On his return to the Zen monastery Mikao Usui bathed, changed his clothes, and requested an audience with the Abbot. During the meeting, while they discussed how he could use his gift of healing, Mikao Usui healed the old Abbot's arthritis.

This miracle represents the cosmic level. Bathing, changing clothes and requesting an audience all represent an initiation. The monastery represents our minds, and the abbot represents our spiritual values and beliefs. Arthritis symbolises becoming frozen in our beliefs—not allowing movement and growth to take place on a spiritual level and preventing us from being in touch with God, our god-self, or our Buddhahood. Healing the Abbot's arthritis symbolises the awakening of Buddhahood.

The Beggar City

Mikao Usui discussed with the Abbot how he could use his gift of healing. Eventually it was decided that Mikao would go to the Beggar City in Kyoto so he could help the poor and destitute to have better lives. He worked there for seven years.

The Beggar City represents a negative state of mind which includes a poverty mentality, doubts and fears. The Beggar City can found within yourself and within others. Each one of us will spend some time in our own Beggar City. Seven years indicates that his experience was a spiritual journey. It may not have actually taken Mikao Usui seven years but seven stages to complete and integrate the lessons learned during this experience. The Beggar City and its young men, I believe, represents the first level of the Healing Buddha mandala which symbolises healing our Yang (positive) energy.

Some versions of the Reiki Story give a description of the Chief of the Beggar City who takes Mikao Usui's clothes away replacing them with rags, allows him only one meal a day and lets him live in a tiny hovel then demands all the money Mikao Usui earns teaching Reiki. In every good fairy tale there is someone wicked who externalises our negative thoughts and feelings. The Beggar Chief, who was so mean to Mikao Usui, stands for those times we place the blame for our poverty and other troubles onto someone else, instead of seeing that we are the creators of our difficulties.

Mikao Usui chose to heal the young men in the Beggar City. They, he believed, healed quicker than the old because they had less mental/emotional problems attached to their ill health. Once he had given them Reiki he sent the young men to the monastery for a new set of clothes, a new name and a job.

Behind each physical illness there is a mental/emotional or sometimes a spiritual reason. The longer someone has an illness the stronger the negative mental/emotional attitudes

12. THE REIKI STORY—ITS ESOTERIC MEANINGS

which support the illness. Louise Hay's book *Heal Your Body* and Annette Noontil's book *The Body is the Barometer of the Soul* give examples of the kind of attitudes at the base of an illness. Reiki can make us feel we can start life anew just like when we put on new clothes, or give ourselves a new name, or when we start a new job. Reiki will help us to let go of old poverty attitudes and take on new positive attitudes. In the east men can represent positive or yang and women can represent negative or yin. Youth is an early stage of life. This segment of the Reiki story can be related to the Healing Buddha mandala with the young men representing the Yaksha Generals and the Guardians of the Ten Directions who in turn represent various aspects of our lives needing healing. Saying that Mikao Usui healed the young men (positive) in the Beggar City (poverty) symbolises turning attitudes around so that they act, not as hardships, but as positive aspects of your life.

Sending the young men to the monastery for new clothes and a new name can also mean Mikao Usui taught Reiki but the Abbot at the monastery gave the initiations. A new job can mean the young men became monks.

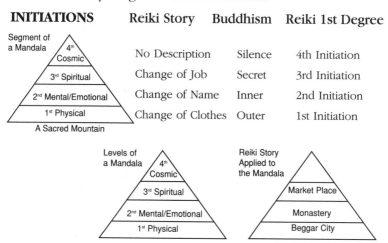

INITIATIONS	**Reiki Story**	**Buddhism**	**Reiki 1st Degree**
No Description		Silence	4th Initiation
Change of Job		Secret	3rd Initiation
Change of Name		Inner	2nd Initiation
Change of Clothes		Outer	1st Initiation

Segment of a Mandala — 4th Cosmic / 3rd Spiritual / 2nd Mental/Emotional / 1st Physical — A Sacred Mountain

Levels of a Mandala — 4th Cosmic / 3rd Spiritual / 2nd Mental/Emotional / 1st Physical

Reiki Story Applied to the Mandala — Market Place / Monastery / Beggar City

One day Mikao Usui realised that he was seeing the same young men again. He asked why they had returned to the Beggar City. Their reply was that it was easier to beg and steal than to change their lives and work for a living.

No matter how enthusiastic we may be about Reiki there will be people we will not be able to help because they do not want to change their lives. Or, we can be like the young men and resist change ourselves. A poor attitude towards life, work and relationships is easier to hold on to in our lives than a positive, active attitude. A positive attitude takes conscious effort to maintain at all times before it becomes second nature. We also can have positive thoughts which we do nothing with—ideas that come into our minds but take no action on. These ideas can return to our awareness several times and each time we will think of a reason why we do not follow the idea through into manifestation—such as: "I can't afford it"; "I don't have the experience or education"; or, "What will people say" and so on.

Deeply upset, some say he fell down with his face in the mud. It was then that Mikao Usui realised that he was healing the body but not the spirit or the mind.

In Japan the expression "he fell down with his face in the mud" would signify that Mikao Usui was deeply ashamed. It also indicates the lowest point of a journey which appears at the bottom point of a mandala. This segment of a mandala is allocated the element Water which, when mixed with the Earth element of a mountain (mandala), turns to mud.

When we first begin using Reiki we usually concentrate on healing the body and are excited when we see a miraculous recovery. We tend not to notice or be concerned with healing the mental/emotional or spiritual levels because they are less noticeable and harder to credit to Reiki and the treatments given. At some time in our Reiki experience we may feel embarrassed or disappointed because our Reiki treatments have not worked on the physical level. We need to practice detachment from the outcome of a Reiki treatment; to remember that we are not doing the healing, that we are channels for the energy and it is the person receiving the treatment who ultimately decides on being healed or not.

Simply replacing poor attitudes with positive ones is not enough. The poor attitudes have to be healed first before work can be done programming positive attitudes. Each cell in our body contains space, memory and intelligence therefore each cell can absorb and remember our positive and negative responses. To overcome the negative responses of your body you need to reprogramme or re-educate the cells. The first level of Reiki, in my opinion, is about re-educating the cells of the body. Healing the body represent 1st Degree Reiki.

The Return to the Monastery

Returning to the monastery Mikao Usui spent time meditating on Reiki and how to use Reiki so that the healing was permanent.

As previously noted a monastery can represent ourselves. Whenever we find ourselves within a Beggar City, either our own or someone else's we can find our way out of that city by going back to that quiet, still, and wise part of ourselves which is usually found during meditation. It also means taking a look at what is going on in our minds, and healing our thoughts. The monastery, where they heal the mind, represents 2nd Degree Reiki.

After a period of meditation Mikao Usui decided that adding the Five Principles to the Reiki would make it more effective.

The Reiki principles are meant to be integrated into the philosopy of the Reiki practitioner, not just written on a fancy piece of paper and displayed on a wall. They are active symbols which are meant to be incorporated within your daily living and into your treatments. Including the Reiki principles into your Reiki treatments enables them to work at a deep unconscious level until they become an innate part of you. The speed in which the Reiki Principles work depends on how often you use them.

The Reiki principles will act like a mirror, showing you where you need to work on yourself. That area of your life will keep coming back, stronger and stronger, until you face it and deal with it in a calm and detached way. Whenever worry, anger or one of the other aspects of the principles turns up in your life the easiest way to achieve that calmness so that you can be objective is to give yourself a Reiki Self-treatment and repeat the Principles to yourself at each hand position.

The Reiki Principles can be used to re-educate the cells of our body. Each cell is a living being and a microcosm of the whole body. Repeating the Five Reiki Principles while holding our hand over the painful areas of the body teaches the cells not to take on either worry or anger; to honour the instructions from their parents, teachers, and elders (the paracrine, endocrine and nervous systems); to work well, efficiently and successfully; and to be in harmony with other cells in the body.

The Exchange

Mikao Usui came to the conclusion that there needed to be an energy exchange so the gift of Reiki would be appreciated.

His decision is reflected in the sutra of the Healing Buddha where the Buddha said that there are people who do not know what it is to make a gift or know what the results of making a gift are and it is in the best interest of all concerned to teach them how to make a gift.

It appears an energy exchange is one of the natural laws of the universe which in Buddhism is "cause and effect" or "karma" and in Christianity is "sowing and reaping". The Reiki story does not say how much or what the exchange is to be. My experience has taught me that it is not what you charge for Reiki that matters but how you feel about that charge or exchange. If you are not totally at peace with the fees you charge for Reiki classes or treatments you will have trouble with them. This may manifest as worry about your income, fear of competition, doubts about overcharging or undercharging, doubts about how much you deserve to receive, and your ability to give and share or you may feel resentful or angry towards others who charge more or less than you. You may receive cheques which bounce; teach people who expect to pay their class fees off very, very slowly; or who, to your annoyance and embarrassment, at the end of a class declare they don't have any money and make no offer to pay.

Whatever someone else may suggest you charge for Reiki, unless you are totally at ease with the exchange you will have difficulty with it, plus you will feel resentful towards that person for engendering the feeling of unease within you. There is a need to approach your Reiki exchange with Zen-like detachment. To do this you need to set an exchange rate that you feel completely happy with then do what Mikao Usui did, meditate and come to a decision about it, an acceptance of it. We all need to reach, and be comfortable with, our own view and understanding of the energy exchange.

Buddhists believe that as long as you owe someone or someone owes you something (karma) you will continue to be reborn (reincarnate) and will be unable to ascend to the higher realms. Therefore you should ensure that not only are all your debts paid but that no-one owes you any debts or favours otherwise you will need to return to this realm once again to collect or pay them.

The energy exchange also relates to the amount of energy or effort you put into doing something. The more effort you put into what you do the greater the results. An example of the energy exchange can be seen when placing Reiki symbols on a cash register in a shop to attract more customers into your shop. More customers mean you will have to expend more energy to deal with them by either working harder or paying wages for more staff.

Presenting Reiki to Others

He also decided that he would not push Reiki on anyone and everyone, but to pass it on to those people who were interested and wanted Reiki in their lives.

Pushing Reiki onto people who are not ready to accept it is a way of trying to set goals for another person's journey. Only the person concerned really knows what their goals in life are and only they can make their journey. Another person cannot do it for them nor can they judge when that person is ready for the journey.

Another aspect of this is that you do not need to consciously push the Reiki energy through yourself or the person receiving it when you give a Reiki treatment. Reiki will flow naturally without having to apply any physical or mental effort to it.

Torch in Daylight

Mikao Usui then began travelling around Japan, from village to village and town to town teaching Reiki.

This part of the story is about teaching Reiki. In the Christian segment of the Reiki Story it is said Mikao Usui came home to Japan–Japan in the Reiki Story can therefore represent yourself (home). A village or town is an energy centre for a district. So this part of the Reiki Story describes 1st Degree Reiki–teaching Reiki to your energy centres (the endocrine or chakra system of the body).

He would stand on a street corner or in the local marketplace with a large lighted torch in daylight. People would laugh at him and point out to him that it was already daylight, and there was no need to carry a lighted torch.

This is an example of standing in your own light, of believing in yourself and in Reiki, no matter how much someone may ridicule you; of "walking your walk, and talking your talk". The marketplace refers to living in the workaday world outside of a monastery. This part of the Reiki story echos the tenth picture in the "Ox Herding Pictures" of Zen Buddhism which demonstrates being able to put into practice all the lessons learned in the monastery while out in the marketplace; of remaining peaceful and joyful no matter what you experience when interacting with the world around you.

On another level the Kanji characters for "Torch in Daylight" appear within the Reiki Master symbol. To me this means that Mikao Usui was actively symbolising the Master symbol as he travelled around Japan. For Reiki Masters this means that we integrate Reiki and the Master symbol so that we can shine our inner light outwards to others. We can stand in the light, not matter how bright, and be a shining example to others of what Reiki is and can be within someone's life. The Buddha Sakyamuni's last words are reputed to be: "Be a Lamp unto yourself."

Teaching Reiki

Usui would reply that if they were interested he could teach them how to have more light, enjoyment and health in their lives. Then Mikao Usui would invite them to go to a nearby temple, either in the afternoon or evening, to listen to him talk about Reiki. He would then wait at the temple and teach Reiki to those who were interested enough to come along to listen to him.

This part of the Reiki story is about teaching 2nd Degree Reiki. In the early part of the Reiki Story Mikao Usui visited various monasteries where they said they only healed the mind. Sitting in the temple and teaching Reiki is about teaching Reiki and the attitudes of enjoyment, health, happiness and light to the mind.

Mikao Usui also gives Reiki Teachers an example of trusting the universe to provide them with students; allowing the students to make up their own minds about who they wish to do their Reiki training with, when and where.

Rebirth to a higher plane is often a central theme of fairy tales and going from teaching Reiki in the Beggar City to teaching it in a temple is an example of transformation or rebirth to a higher form of existence. It may also indicate that Mikao Usui had reach a level where he could both teach and initiate students.

Conclusion

The Reiki Story has a happy ending, providing us with a very positive template for the future of Reiki. Presently there is a lot of mistrust, discord and competitiveness between Reiki Masters around the world which would indicate that many of us are still operating in our Beggar Cities or, in other words, we have not completed the work of 1st Degree Reiki yet. Once we have moved through this period, have integrated the lessons, balanced our energies and reprogrammed our cells with the principles, and can shine our inner light to the world we will be able to take Reiki into the market place with enjoyment, in peace and harmony as living examples of the benefits of Reiki.

The Reiki Story is, I believe, one of the sacred symbols of Reiki. It may in fact be the most important symbol of Reiki because the symbolism contained within the story has been so deeply and cleverly hidden within a story about Mikao Usui.

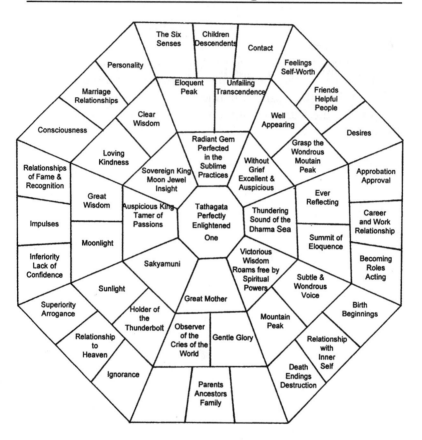

Chapter 13

THE HEALING BUDDHA MANDALA AND REIKI

*N*o-one in the Reiki community, as far as I am
aware, has applied Reiki to the Healing Buddha
mandala before; therefore this chapter is based
purely on my own experience of Reiki and my own interpretation of the Healing Buddha Mandala.

The Healing Buddha mandala, I believe, is an illustration
of the Reiki energy, as well as being a description of the best
way to work with Reiki. It also illustrates the journey that the
Reiki energy takes you on when you become initiated to
Reiki. Each step of the journey is represented by the figure of
a being—either a Buddha, Goddess, Bodhisattva, Guardian
or General—signifying that the journey is a personal one.

When you are initiated
to Reiki you step into the
Healing Buddha mandala
which is a journey that
takes you to your thoughts
and feelings, your desires
and illusions, allows you to
revisit your past, and to
take a new look at your
relationships. You travel to
parts of yourself you have
never known before and it
enables you to look in new
ways at the parts you are
familiar with. It allows you to express your true Self and to
become a balanced and fully integrated person.

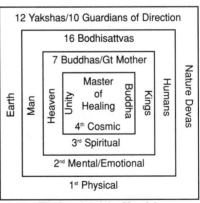

The Levels of the Mandala

The Reiki Degrees in Relation to the Mandala

The mandala is divided into seven active sections (the seven male Buddhas) and one passive section (the one female Goddess). Therefore I believe each Reiki Degree has seven steps (the seven male Buddhas). When each of the seven steps has been completed there is a gift (bestowed by the female Goddess), which signifies acknowledgement of your progress. The Goddess can also represent times of initiation.

Each of the eight sections of the mandala on the third level appear to act as the underlying theme or influence for the first two levels of the mandala and then becomes the main influence at the third level. Although these stages of the mandala are not taught in Reiki classes they still, I believe, have an influence on the Reiki student who presently works through them unconsciously. In Buddhism the student is taught to work through the stages of the mandala consciously, with an understanding of the ultimate aim of the mandala, and with longer contact with and regular guidance from the Master/Lama/Guru/Abbot.

In the west the speed in which people move from one Reiki degree to the next has increased until now some people travel through the Reiki degrees, from 1st to 3rd, in sixteen hours during one weekend or even faster by doing all three degrees in one day. I am of the opinion that no matter how fast or slow a person moves through the Reiki system they still have to go through the steps and process of the Healing Buddha's mandala. They may have a certificate that affirms they are 3rd Degree Reiki, but until they have done the work of the three levels of the mandala they will not be "energetically" 3rd Degree Reiki. The old Greek legend of Icarus who flew too close to the sun (spiritual journey) so that the wax on his wings (not enough preparation) melted

and he fell into the sea (despair) and drowned is about someone who tries rushing through their spiritual journey without
doing the correct preparation. In his case the result was
despair and death. There are a number of legends world-
wide about the folly of trying to rush through a spiritual journey without doing the work and preparation first. I believe
we need to take heed of those stories.

A person who has completed the seven steps of all three
degrees then moves on to 4th Degree and becomes a Master
of Healing. This step is what is known within Buddhism as
"Enlightenment". The process is described in the Reiki Story
as the time when Mikao Usui was hit by light, saw bubbles
of many colours and knew and understood the whole system
of Reiki.

Entering the Mandala

Entry into a mandala is through the East Gate. Manjusri,
one of the two Bodhisattvas who sit in the eastern section of
the mandala, has promised to tell everyone who belongs to a
"good family" about the Healing Buddha, even if he has to
shout in their ear while they are asleep. I believe that "good
family" means people who have an innate goodness in their
basic nature which can be developed with practice.

The Guardian King who sits at the Eastern Gate is passive, which means that he won't stop anyone who has heard
about Reiki and wants to do Reiki from entering the mandala.
This is supported by the fact that anyone regardless of race,
religion, sex or age can be attuned to Reiki. However the
Guardian Kings at the other gates—South, West and North—
are active and therefore, I believe can, and do prevent, people from entering the higher levels of the energy of Reiki.
This is supported by many people who describe the energy
working coincidentally or mysteriously in their lives just prior

to doing their second and third degree classes—indicating to me the Reiki practitioner's readiness to receive the next initiation. Another way, I believe, of not being allowed to enter the higher levels of Reiki is by being attracted to Reiki Masters who do less than four initiations during a First Degree Reiki class.

First Degree Initiations	Guardian King	Innate Quality
First	East	Goodness
Second	South	Generosity
Third	West	Compassion
Fourth	North	Excellence

THE THREE PATHWAYS

The first three levels of the mandala are three separate pathways or journeys. The first level is the Homeless Pathway which means leaving behind all those actions, relationships and attitudes that you are comfortable with, and that help you to define your role in your community and with your friends and family. Travelling along this pathway means letting go of familiar habits, actions, responses, and relationships which do not benefit you. Developing your innate goodness, learning not to be judgmental and becoming more observant of your behaviour will help you to successfully travel this pathway.

The second pathway is known as the Bodhisattva Pathway. On this journey you learn to change your thoughts and feelings so they benefit and bless you. Healing these energies brings enthusiasm and enjoyment to living as well as self-worth. Developing your generosity towards, and compassion for, others will help you move along this pathway.

The third journey is the Pathway of the Kings or Buddhas. A king is the symbolic link between heavenly and earthly power. This pathway teaches you how to make this link—to bring together thoughts and actions so that they act as one force. A king is also a symbol of rulership over unconscious urges. Continuing to exercise compassion and generosity as well as recognising when you create karma and learning how to stop creating karma allows you to travel this pathway. When you develop all three levels to a point of excellence you will reach fourth level which is Enlightenment.

The First Level of the Mandala = 1st Degree Reiki

The outer circle of the Mandala containing the Yaksha Generals and Guardians of the Ten Directions is, I believe, the equivalent to 1st Degree Reiki. This level is divided into twenty two sections. One section, East, is passive and represents your entry into Reiki; the other 21 sections denote the active steps or work to be done to master 1st Degree Reiki. Each section is personified by either a Yaksha General symbolising how our body responds or acts, or one of the Guardians of the Ten Directions representing our relationships. Each of these personifications has a partner. The partner of each Yaksha General is an animal and each of the Guardians of the Ten Directions has a female partner. As each General and Guardian is a symbol they have multiple meanings. As representatives of time (Generals) and place (Guardians) their partners represent balance in these areas. One of the functions of Reiki, in my opinion, is to bring time and place into balance so that the practitioner is in the "right time and right place" each day. This process begins at the first level of Reiki. I also think that the animals represent parts of our bodies and the Yaksha Generals represent the parts of our brain which control or are responsible for that body part.

Another aspect of the Generals and Guardians is to represent the different conditions of our lives that need to be healed so that our lives will be more harmonious and bal-

179

anced. In the Healing Buddha sutras the Yaksha Generals have been treated as a group. Although they have been individually named their individual characteristics have not, nor have the animals they are associated with been named. J W de Visor in *Ancient Buddhism in Japan* does attempt to relate the Generals to time and direction. Because the number 12 can be related to the "12 causes of suffering" I have applied those 12 causes to the 12 Yaksha Generals. The Guardians of the 10 Directions also tend to be written about as a "group" and not as the kinds of relationships they represent or guard. I have applied the Feng Shui relationships as shown on a Ba Gua, to these Guardians.

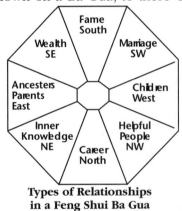

Types of Relationships in a Feng Shui Ba Gua

I believe it is not unreasonable to allocate these aspects of the Ba Gua to the Guardians of the 10 Directions of a mandala because the influence of the Ba Gua underlies the mandala which has evolved from the Ba Gua. Buddhism and Taoism exchanged many concepts when they met in China.

I have therefore applied the following relationships to the Guardians of the Ten Directions:

East	Relationships with Ancestors/Parents/Elders/Lineage
South East	Relationships with Heaven/God/Universe/Luck/Fates/Wealth
South	Relationships based on Fame/Recognition/Reputation
South West	Marriage and Partnership Relationships
West	Relationships with Children/Siblings
North	Relationships with Workmates/Colleagues/Employers/Employees
North East	Relationship with your Self

13. The Healing Buddha Mandala and Reiki

In the Healing Buddha Land there is no "above" and "below" therefore the Guardians of these two directions become Yaksha Generals. The Twelve Yaksha Generals when related (by me) to the 12 causes of suffering are:

1. Kumbhira	=	Ignorance	6. Sanila	=	Contact
Above	=	Superiority/Arrogance	7. Indra	=	Feelings
Below	=	Inferiority/Lack	8. Pajra	=	Desires
2. Vajra	=	Impulses	9. Makura	=	Approbation
3. Mihira	=	Consciousness	10. Kinnara	=	Becoming
4. Anila	=	Personality	11. Catura	=	Birth
5. Manila	=	The Six Senses	12. Vikarala	=	Death

How our bodies respond to these causes can be represented by the animals which accompany the Generals. Buddhists sometimes describe the mind as an animal to explain the behaviour of thoughts by saying, for instance, the monkey mind jumps between the branches of fame and fortune, and the wild horse mind gallops through the fields of desire. Some pictures of the Yaksha Generals show each of them with an animal from the Chinese Zodiac. A description of one of these zodiac animals often includes their attitude and behaviour. For instance the Rat can represent aggression, restlessness, anxiety and nervousness. The Yaksha Generals also, in my opinion, indicate our human awareness while their animal partners represent our basic animal instincts and reactions; those times when we lash out or respond without thinking. In the Old Testament it tells us that mankind has dominion over the animal kingdom. For me that does not mean we are boss over the animals that cohabit this planet with us but that we can control and rise above the animal nature which resides within us. Each of the Generals is shown either astride or above their animal partner, implying that they have tamed the animal nature of their minds and bodies.

The Generals and Guardians personify those behaviours and attitudes which can cause difficulties in our lives. The mandala tells us that we need to bring these behaviours and attitudes into harmony and balance. At the first level each of the eight segments of the mandala is divided into three parts (except East). Three represents positive, negative and neutral. These three parts indicate that our relationship and how we deal with the world can be either positive, negative or neutral. The optimum is to be neutral—not positive, not negative—not this, not that—not good, not bad but in between.

HATE	COMPASSION/KINDNESS	LOVE		
(negative)	(neutral)	(positive)	Yang	Yin
(Yin)	(Yin/Yang)	(Yang)		
(- polarity)	(0 polarity)	(+ polarity)	**Yin/Yang Symbol**	

At first glance neutral appears to be a situation where there is no positive and no negative but this is not what neutral is. Neutral is when the two energies of positive and negative are acting together as one energy. This is represented by the Yin/Yang symbol which show negative and positive being held together within a circle. Neutral therefore does not mean nothing—it means the point where positive and negative are exactly the same, where there is no polarity between the two, yet it does not mean they cancel each other out. Instead together they become a new unit. Reiki, which is non-polar energy, helps us to stop swinging from positive to negative and back again and enables us to stay centred between the two polarities.

During each of the 21 days on the mountain Mikao Usui threw away a stone until he finally saw the light just before dawn. Stones symbolise the behaviours and problems that are personified by the Generals and Guardians. Each day we do a Reiki self-treatment we also throw away a stone.

13. The Healing Buddha Mandala and Reiki

The Second Level of the Mandala = Reiki 2nd Degree

On the mandala the second level is personified by Bodhisattvas (enlightened beings) each of whom is the leader of a family or energy group which needs to be brought together in harmony so they work towards one goal rather than conflicting goals. As Bodhisattvas they have vowed to put their own needs aside and act to benefit all sentient beings. I believe that 2nd Degree Reiki was originally taught over 14 stages with each stage made up of a programme based on one of the Bodhisattva families shown on the mandala.

The second level of the mandala is often held to be very secret and it is probably because of this that 2nd Degree of Reiki has a great deal of secrecy surrounding it. This is the feminine level of the mandala and because so much secrecy has always surrounded a woman's rites of passage through life this level is held to be secret. It is the level which explores our inner world which holds our thoughts, feelings, fears, doubts, dreams, hopes and secrets. This level is therefore about bringing your Yin/negative/passive/feminine energy into balance. In Buddhism it is called the Bodhisattva Pathway. At this level there are also seven steps but this time each step is divided in half to form 14 sections - Heart and Mind—which can be related to Second Degree Reiki, often called the Mental/Emotional level of Reiki. This division of the second level of the mandala can also symbolise the idea that feminine energy has two sides to it—one vengeful (witch), the other beneficial (goddess). This level also focuses on developing a wish to help all sentient beings and accumulating merit.

The Third Level of the Mandala = 3rd Degree Reiki

The third level of the Mandala has eight sections—seven male Buddhas and the Great Mother/Vajradhara. I think that originally a Reiki Master took seven years to complete their training, working with each of the seven Healing Buddhas for a year. This work, according to the sutra for the Seven Healing Buddhas, probably included: repeating the name of the Buddha, his vows, and any spiritual formulae pertaining to that Buddha three to six times each day; visualising the Buddha's pure land during meditation; plus other exercises which were passed on orally at the time of initiation. It seems to me that the generosity and compassion that was developed at the second level is now tempered with thoughts of loving kindness, peace and joy; The Master can access his field of accumulated merit from which all desires are fulfilled. The vows of each of the Buddhas indicate the kind of merits that have been accumulated and which can be accessed.

The Fourth Level of the Mandala = Enlightenment (no Reiki equivalent)

The Reiki story tells of Mikao Usui being hit by light and seeing lots of coloured bubbles, symbols and understanding the whole system of Reiki while on top of the mountain, indicating to me that he reached enlightenment and the fourth level of the mandala. As Master of Healing he would've been in complete "oneness" with the universal healing energies.

In Buddhism there appears to be four initiations at this level of a mandala. The first three are bestowed by a Master while the fourth is said to be innate in that it happens of its own accord and is not given by anyone. This "automatic" initiation, when you become your own Master, is known as "Innate Joy" in Tantric Buddhism. I have no doubt therefore, that when a Reiki Master has truly mastered all aspects of Reiki they will experience a spontaneous initiation. However. Keith Dowman in *Sky Dancer* says that uncontrolled mental chatter, deeply held thoughts which originate from childhood, and rigid beliefs will prevent you from experiencing this initiation.

WORKING THROUGH THE MANDALA
Level 1 - Twenty One Day Programme

I believe 1st Degree Reiki was a 21 day programme spent understanding relationships and the causes of the problems within a relationship and then giving and receiving Reiki to heal the relationships and causes afflicting the life of the person participating in the programme. The participants would live in a monastery for the whole 21 day period so they could focus fully on the programme. At present Reiki practitioners have to go through this cycle of the energy on their own, away from the class, and without the knowledge of what they will go through. In my opinion, even if we are not taught the seven stages of each Degree we still experience them, and are often presented with the relationships we have difficulty with and move on when we recognise and let go of the problems which have made our relationships difficult. Because we are not taught the individual steps of the first level of the mandala we often do not understand why difficulties arise in our life and believe Reiki is not working. If there are difficulties Reiki can make them come to the surface like a boil, which can then be lanced and healed.

First Degree Reiki, as far as I am concerned, is about healing our outer life and its impact on our bodies, which is reflected in our actions, reactions and relationships, so that we can look at the world outside of ourselves in a meaningful and positive way. This means looking at both the negative and positive aspects of a relationship then bringing the two sides together so they form a new way of dealing with the relationship which is honest and beneficial. It is learning to make relationships work for you and not against you.

I worked through 1st Degree Reiki again by doing a 21

day Reiki programme on myself. I collected 21 white stones from the beach at Gore Bay in the South Island of New Zealand, and with a blue felt-tip pen wrote on each stone what I wanted healed.

Day 1:	Misconceptions
Day 2:	Relationship with Heaven
Day 3:	Arrogance
Day 4:	Inferiority
Day 5:	Impulses
Day 6:	Relationship with the Famous
Day 7:	Consciousness
Day 8:	Marriage/Partner Relationship
Day 9:	Personality
Day 10:	The Six Senses
Day 11:	Relationship with Children
Day 12:	Contact
Day 13:	Feelings
Day 14:	Relationship with Friends
Day 15:	Desires
Day 16:	Approbation
Day 17:	Career and Work
Day 18:	Becoming
Day 19:	Birth
Day 20:	Relationship with Yourself
Day 21:	Death

At the beginning of each self treatment I said: Let this Reiki treatment heal my... . I then said the attitude or relationship for that day. Then I gave myself a Reiki treatment using the 12 hand positions for a self treatment. At each hand position I said the intent again and chanted to myself all Five Reiki Principles at least three times or more. At the end of the treatment I turned the stone over (I didn't throw the stones away because I wanted to use them again). Originally I only used the intent at the begining of the treatment. A friend did this 21 day programme and she reaffirmed the intent at each hand position because she felt doing so made reprogramming the body more effective. I tried her way and found I had to agree with her. I have also treated clients with this programme and I find it an excellent way of focusing on the person I am treating. A number of Reiki people have done this programme and found it to be very beneficial.

1st Level Step One

RELATIONSHIP:

God/Universe/Heaven or Luck/Fate (In Feng Shui this point of the Ba Gua also includes your relationship with money—indicating that if you heal your relationship with God you will heal your relationship with money.)

CAUSE OF PROBLEMS:

Ignorance—misconceptions about the laws of life. (This is not "lack of knowledge" but wrong/incorrect beliefs).

Arrogance—believing you are above/beyond the laws of life. (This includes using God's name to have authority over others).

1st Level Step Two

RELATIONSHIP:

With people we judge to have more fame, recognition, influence, power, or money etc, than ourselves.

CAUSE OF PROBLEMS:

Inferiority—feel we are not important or of less value than someone else.

Impulses—being influenced by the latest person you've met or latest book read, the latest idea or fashion, etc.— impulsively rushing from one thing to another, changing your mind with each new thing that catches your attention.

1st Level Step Three

RELATIONSHIP:

Marriage/Intimate Partnerships

CAUSE OF PROBLEMS:

Consciousness ie: Ego = I. Always putting yourself first without considering the consequences your actions will have on other people. Also means the need to name things—ie this is mine, that is your's.

Personality—the conditioning received and behaviour learnt which can interfere with or block your intimate relationships such as sexual injunctions learned during the process of growing up.

1st Level Step Four

RELATIONSHIP:

Children/Grandchildren/Siblings

CAUSE OF PROBLEMS:

The six senses—sight, sound, touch, taste, smell, intuition. Many of us do not use our senses efficiently enough—we don't listen when we should, take no notice of taste or smell, or have little regard for the messages our intuition sends us.

Contact—how you relate to someone through the senses ie: are you a "touch" person or a "sound" person; do you remember someone by their perfume or by the meal you ate together, or what they wore?

1st Level Step Five

RELATIONSHIP: Friends and helpful people

CAUSE OF PROBLEMS:

Feelings—being easily hurt by, or overly sensitive to deeds and words or the reverse, insensitive or callous towards other people's feelings.

Desires—wants which conflict with someone else's needs. Always wanting and never being satisfied with what you already have.

1st Level Step Six

RELATIONSHIP:

Career and Work relationships

CAUSE OF PROBLEMS:

Approbation—seeking constant approval.

Becoming—changing your behaviour for different people ie: you behave one way with your boss, another with people who report to you, another way towards your peers, yet another way with customers, and so on.

1st Level Step Seven

RELATIONSHIP:

With yourself—often called our Inner Self because we hide our true self from the rest of the world.

CAUSE OF PROBLEMS:

Birth—dreams, hopes, intents, wishes, talents you are born with. Starting something new, often before completing your previous project/job. Also can apply to your reason for being born to this life, your purpose as well as the physical trauma you went through being born, which was your initial experience of this life.

Death—destroying your dreams, hopes, intents, wishes, talents. Losing the enthusiasm to complete something you started. Talking yourself out of (or being talked out of) trying something new. Also can apply to your fear of death and how you intend to die.

1st Level—Step Eight—The Gift

RELATIONSHIP:

Parents, Elders, Ancestors

The eighth step of the mandala is a gift. If all the work of the first seven steps is done then the eighth step happens automatically without any effort. If your relationship with your parents is difficult/hurtful it can be the hardest relationship to experience. It is the relationship which acts like a blueprint for all our other relationships. The mandala deals with this relationship by healing all the other relationships and their causes in your life first so that when you reach the point of healing your relationship with your parents a great deal of it will have healed of its own accord.

Second Level —14 Months Programme

Not enough material is available about the second level of the mandala so I have been unable to work through each of the steps of this area of the Healing Buddha mandala.

It is my opinion that 2nd Degree Reiki was originally a 14 months' programme with each month being a lunar month rather than a calendar month. The second level of the mandala is aligned to the cycle of the moon and many Buddhist ceremonies are based on the phases of the moon. I do not know what the actual programme would have been. My guess is that it was based on the Buddhist programme for becoming a Bodhisattva.

Unfortunately there are no records in English, that I know of, for all the Bodhisattva families for the Healing Buddha mandala. I used Bodhisattva families from other mandalas. Two appear in the *Buddhist Tantras*—they are the 37 Natures of Enlightenment and the Mt Meru Mandala. The Diamond family appears in the book *Indo-Tibetan Buddhism Vol 1*. Although there are 37 members of a Bodhisattva family I found that only 28 members (almost a lunar month) need healing. I believe a Bodhisattva family consists of:

The Leader of the Family—appears on the Healing Buddha's mandala. The leader does not need Reiki treatments to be 'healed' as it represents the whole family when it is healed and working together in harmony and for your benefit.

Eight Goddesses—these Goddesses also do not require healing. They represent parts of you which are innate and perfect. However they cannot express themselves properly if their family is not working in harmony and for your benefit. If your Bodhisattva family is in confusion or conflict then the goddesses can become vengeful witches. When the family is healed and in harmony they becomes beautiful goddesses who work for your benefit. These Goddesses also protect the family and their permission must be obtained before entering the Bodhisattva family.

Four Doormen—who sit at the four directions of East, South, West and North. They guard the gateways into the family. They must be healed first before going further into the family—otherwise they will stop you in some way. They represent the conditions which activate the family—open the doors to the family—the passwords and activities which open or close the doors. For example, some Doormen open the door when you take on a 'burden' (because your family likes being a martyr), some close the door when you are asked to help someone (because your family does not like responsibility).

Eight Guardians—who also sit at the four directions of East, South, West and North, as well as the four intermediary directions of South East, South West, North West and North East. They need to be healed next. They act as Guardians and when healed support, encourage, help and protect the family in its activities.

16 Bodhisattvas who consist of:

• **The Seven Limbs** • **The Four Faculties** • **The Five Natures**

These appear to be ways of thinking, feeling and expressing ourselves. They need healing so that they work together and help you to be happy and fortunate.

191

Myself and several friends worked through the Bodhisattva families that I was able to discover and found it an interesting experience. Firstly we needed to get permission from one of the eight Goddesses and had to have an initiation before we could enter the family which was followed by a twenty-eight day healing programme using the second degree Reiki symbols and the Mental/Emotional technique on the head, throat and heart with the following intent: *"Let this Reiki treatment heal my (then say the name of the Doorman, Guardian, or Bodhisattva) so it becomes a friend of all living beings and ensures there is happiness and good fortune for all living beings"*.

Both the first and second level programmes created a lot of vivid dreams. It seemed to me they acted as new intents which had to be processed at dream level to enable both our inner and outer worlds to be altered. Dreaming is said to play an important role in the attainment of enlightenment because dreams originate from the total person. I find myself now being more at ease with people, less likely to get picked up and carried away by other people's dramas, less worried about the future and my intuition is clearer and more reliable. However, I recommend that a Reiki programme based on the Bodhisattva families is accompanied by expert guidance and counselling that includes explanations of dreams and discussion of the mental and emotional aspects that emerge.

Heart—Accumulating Merit

In Buddhism an important aspect of Bodhisattva training is to encourage the qualities of generosity and service to others. The aim is to build up merit or as some would say in the west, "Brownie points". The Reiki Story tells us about an energy exchange—each time you give something or do something there is an exchange of energy—not always a monetary one—in other words for each good turn you do for others you gain merit. In the Healing Buddha sutra the Buddha points out that many people do not understand this philosophy and need to be taught this by making them pay with money or goods for the services you do for them. Their payment will earn them merit. Begrudging the payment will earn less merit than paying with goodwill, therefore it is recommended that you bless your money and all payments you make for any service you receive. When you have acquired enough merit you can then move on to the third level of the mandala. Merit can be gained by being generous with how you speak or think about people, including yourself. Often we begrudge other people their good fortune or are fearful of our own.

In Reiki we can gain merit by giving Reiki treatments and doing Distance Healing. It does not matter if we charge for these services or not what matters is how we feel about giving the treatments. We gain more merit if we can give selflessly and without thought of reward (do not focus on an outcome). When attending a Reiki Support Group you receive one treatment and give several. All the treatments you give gain you merit. Unfortunately I have attended Support Groups where someone has received a Reiki treatment (usually the first one) and then left without helping to give Reiki treatments to the rest of the group. Giving Reiki treatments allows us to develop our innate generosity. Closing our eyes and allowing the Reiki to flow through us without any thought of the consequences or rewards helps us let go of selfishness. After a while you will find it easy to express your generosity and willingness to help others in other areas of your life. As you begin to get praise and thanks for your actions, cards saying thank you, and gifts of appreciation you will be able to accept them graciously because you will know you have done the work and you deserve the acclaim. You will also find it easier to praise others. The consequence is an increase in your self-worth and self-esteem because you will recognise that the praise and appreciation is honest and deserved. When your mental/emotional merit field reaches the point of overflowing into your physical life in this way it is time to move on to the third level of Reiki. Be warned that anger can destroy aeons of accumulated merit, hence we learn not to allow anger to arise at the first level of the mandala.

Mind - Purifying Obscurations

According to Pabongka Rinpoche in *Liberation in the Palm of Your Hand,* another important practice for someone on the Bodhisattva pathway is to purify your obscurations—those dull, indefinite, hidden, unnoticed, gloomy, confusing, doubtful and not clearly expressed thoughts and feelings—so they become clean, clear and bright. The name of the Distance Healing symbol tells us "This person righteously adjusts their thoughts and feelings" so this symbol can be used each day to purify your obscurations. This requires taking note of when you start getting confused, have doubts, or are not thinking clearly. Then you can:

1. Draw a large Distance Healing symbol in front of you and step into it and say the name of the symbol three times. Then ask for clarity about the particular thought, idea or emotion that is not clear. Step back out of the symbol when your thoughts or emotion becomes peaceful.

2. Mentally draw the Distance Healing symbol and imagine it going into the top of your head bringing order to the chaos that is going on in your mind.

3. When I get mean, unhappy or angry thoughts I say, "Begone unpleasant thought. This is a Royal Command!" Then I draw the Power symbol and say its name three times.

13. THE HEALING BUDDHA MANDALA AND REIKI

Third Level—7 Year Programme

I have found little within English versions of Buddhist literature which describes this level clearly. The three levels are sometimes referred to as the Outer (1st), the Inner (2nd) and the Secret (3rd) levels. When a practitioner reached this level of the mandala they would have had a clear understanding of the esoteric language (sometimes called Twilight Language) which is used when writing about this level. If they did not understand the language they would not have been accepted for the training that is encompassed within this stage of the mandala.

I think the hand mudras of the Healing Buddhas are an indication of a practitioner's progress through the third level of the mandala.

1st Year–Buddha Sakyamuni—this, I think, means that the first year was spent as a student learning Buddhist theology and practising the techniques used when progressing through the third level of a mandala.

2nd to 4th Years—First three Healing Buddhas—each of these Buddhas hold their right hands in the mudra for teaching while their left hands are in the meditation gesture—signifying they can teach the laws of the mandala. This may mean the practitioner was able to teach students the first level of the mandala during his second year of training, then the first and second levels during his third year, and by the end of his fourth year he would be able to teach all three levels of the mandala.

5th Year–Fourth Healing Buddha—holds both hands in the meditation mudra which indicates the fifth year of training was a year of meditation. The name of the Fourth Healing Buddha's Pure Land would indicate that this year was the time when the student reached a state of excellence in his Healing Buddha practices.

It is interesting to note that in the Reiki Story it is said

Mikao Usui taught the young men in the Beggar City about Reiki then sent them to the monastery for a change of clothes, new name and new job - all being esoterical references to initiations. When he left the Beggar City he returned to the monastery to meditate. This may mean Usui went through this seven year training or the Reiki story was originally about someone else who did.

6th and 7th Years–Fifth and Sixth Healing Buddhas— These two Healing Buddhas hold their right hands in the blessing mudra and their left hands in meditation, which I have assumed means they can give initiations.

At the end of the Reiki story Mikao Usui, after telling people about Reiki, would go to the nearby temple and wait for those people who wanted to know more about Reiki, indicating that Mikao Usui could both teach and initiate people to Reiki. It may mean the Reiki story comes from an older story—not from Mikao Usui or Chujiro Hayashi, but perhaps Japanese Buddhism where it was used to explain the journey through the Healing Buddha mandala.

The third level of the mandala indicates that on reaching 3rd Degree Reiki there is still a lot of work to do—seven years or more. It appears that the 3rd Degree Reiki initiation does not make us Reiki Masters but gives us permission to become Reiki Masters.

Each of the Healing Buddhas who reside at the third level of the mandala has a Pure Land and in each of these lands are bathing pools. According to Pabongka Rinpoche in *Liberation in the Palm of Your Hand,* the bathing in these Pure Land pools is done by visualisation rather than actual bathing. Usui's techniques, Ken Yoku (Dry Bathing) and Jyoshin Kokyuho (Cleansing spirit, heart and mind breathing method) presently taught by Frank Arjava Petter, are excellent ways of doing this kind of bathing. The Healing Buddha sutra instructs us, at this level, to bathe three times a day and make the images of the seven Healing Buddhas. Because the Buddha Sakyamuni calls all the Healing Buddhas together at one time, and also because each of the six Healing Buddhas at the third level of the mandala is an aspect of the Master of Healing, I assume the Reiki Master symbol is the image for all the Healing Buddhas at the third level—remembering that the fourth level where the Master of Healing resides is void and does not contain symbols.

I am still working through this level and have not yet found a way that is as instantly satisfying or as noticeable effective as the 21 Day programme or Bodhisattva Family programmes were, however I realise that the programme could take seven years so the effects may be less instantly observable. Here is a method I do enjoy using:

> Three times a day, begin by dry bathing (Ken Yoku), then do the cleansing spirit, heart and mind breathing method (Jyoshin Kokyuho) for 20 minutes and finish by placing your hands on your heart/chest area and drawing the Reiki Master symbol seven times and saying its name three times each time you draw the symbol.

Another aspect of the third level of the mandala appears to be ensuring you do not create karma. On the second level the lesson is to give without regret, while on the third level this becomes giving without expectation. This is done by observing when you believe someone "owes" you something. This may be a favour, money, or revenge which is often accompanied by feelings and thoughts justifying why something is owed to you. When you have a belief that someone "owes" you something then you are creating karma. When you do someone a favour (when you benefit a sentient being) instead of accumulating that favour and expecting it to be repaid to you by that person sometime in the future add that good deed to your merit field. Visualise yourself hanging it as a beautiful gemstone on a tree with other gemstones so that it becomes a wish-fulfilling tree. Then when you send out a wish visualise God or an Angel plucking one of the gems from your wish-fulfilling tree and giving it to you.

Trying to work through the various levels of the Healing Buddha mandala has been very interesting. The journey suggests we should be doing more Reiki not less as we move through the levels of Reiki. I am aware that how I worked through the mandala is probably not at all like the way the ancient monks of the Healing Buddha did the work. It is my hope that one day the commentaries (explanations written by monks of earlier ages) associated with the Healing Buddha sutras are translated into English as these, I believe, will give us an even greater insight and understanding of this healing energy we call Reiki.

Bibliography

Anesaki, M. *Buddhist Art*. London: John Murray, 1916.

Anesaki, M. *Buddhist. Art in its Relation to Buddhist Ideals with Special Reference to Buddhism in Japan*. London: John Murray, 1916.

Barnard, Christiann and Illman, John, eds. *The Body Machine*. London: Hamlyn.

Basket, Mary. W. *Footprints of Buddha*. Philadelphia: Philadelphia Museum of Art, 1980.

Bechert, Heinz and Gombrich, Richard, eds. *The World of Buddhism*. London: Thames & Hudson.

Bettelheim, Bruno. *The Uses of Enchantment; The Meaning and Importance of Fairy Tales*. London: Thames & Hudson, 1976.

Bharanti, Agehananda. *The Tantric Tradition*. London: Rider, 1965.

Brinbaum, Raoul *The Healing Buddha*. Boulder: Shambala, 1979.

Bova, Ben. *The Beauty of Light*. New York: Wiley.

Brown, Fran. *Living Reiki Takata's Teachings*. Liferythym, 1992.

Baynes, Cary F. trans. *I Ching or Book of Changes, Richard Wilhelm Translation*. Arkana: Penguin, 1989.

Cady, Duff. *Reiki Returns to Hawayo Takata's House*. William Lee Rand ed. The Reiki News, Fall, 1998.

Campbell, Joseph. *Oriental Mythology: The Masks of God*. Arkana: Penguin, 1976.

Chuen, Lam Kam. *The Feng Shui Handbook*. Gaia Books, 1995.

Cleary, Thomas. *The Secret of the Golden Flower*. San Francisco: Harper, 1991.

Cooper, J.C. *Symbolism: The Universal Language*. Aquarian Press, 1982.

Dalai Lama. *A Flash of Lightning in the Dark of Night: A Guide to the Bodhisattva's Way of Life*. Boston & London: Shambala Dragon Editions, 1994.

Dayal, Har. *The Bodhisattva Doctine in Buddhist Sanskrit Literature*. Dehli: Motil Banarsidass, 1978.

DeGroot, J.J.M. *Le Code du Mahayana en Chine*. Amsterdam: Verandeligen der Koninklijke Akademie Van Wetenschappen.

Dowman, Keith. *Sky Dancer, the Secret Life and Songs of the Lady Yeshe Tsogyel*. London: Routledge & Keegan Paul, 1984.

Earhart, A. Byron. *A Religious Study of the Mount Haguro Sect of Shugendo*. Tokyo: Sophia UP.

Elaide, Mircea. *Symbolism, the Sacred, and the Arts*. Ed. Diane Apostalos-Capadona. New York: Continuum, 1992.

Getty, Alice. *The Gods of Northern Buddhism*. USA/Japan: Tuttle.

Guenther, Herbert V. *The Life and Teaching of Naropa*. Boston: Shambala, 1995.

Gyatso, Geshe Kelsang. *Great Treasury of Merit*. London: Tharpa, 1992.

Henshall, Kenneth G. *A Guide to Remembering Japanese Characters*. USA/Japan: Tuttle.

Houston, Jean. *The Hero and the Goddess*. New York: Ballantine, 1992.

Humphreys, Christmas. *A Popular Dictionary of Buddhism*. London: Curzon, 1984.

Ikeda, Daisaku. *The Living Buddha: An Interpretative Biography*. Trans. Burton Watson. Weatherhill, 1976.

International Society for Educational Information, Inc. *The Japanese Emperor through History.*

Jayne, Walter Addison. *The Healing Gods of Ancient Civilization.* New Haven: Yale UP, 1979.

Jichen, Li. *The Realm of Tibetan Buddhism.* Photos: Gu Shoukang and Kang Song. Eds. Xiao Shiling and An Chungyang. Trans. Wang Wenjiong. UBS Publishers' Distributors Ltd.

Jordon, Michaael. *Encyclopedia of the Gods.* London: Kyle Cathie.

Kashiwaahara, Yusen and Sonoda, Koyu, eds. *Shapers of Japanese Buddhism.* Tokyo: Kosei, 1994.

Kidder, J. Edward Jr. *Japanese Temples.* London: Thames & Hudson.

Kohn, Michael H. Trans. *The Shambala Dictionary of Buddhism and Zen.* Boston: Shambala, 1991.

Kornfield, Jack. *A Path with Heart.* New York: Bantam, 1993.

Leeming, David and Page, Jake. *Myths of the Female Divine Goddess.* New York: Oxford UP, 1994.

Lessing, F. D. and Wayman, A. *Introduction to the Buddhist Tantric Systems.* Dehli: Motilal Banarsidass, 1968.

Malalasekera, G.P., ed. *Encyclopedia of Buddhism,* Vo. I. Government of Ceylon, 1961.

Miller, Roy Andrew. *The Footprints of Buddha: An Eight-century Old Japanese Poetic Sequence.* New Haven: American Oriental Society, 1975.

Milner, Kathleen. *Reiki and Other Rays of Touch Healing.* The Healing Arts Series of Kathleen Ann Milner, 1993.

Mochizuki, Toshitaka. *Iyashi No Te (Healing Hands).*

Moore, Steve. *The Trigrams of Han—Inner Structures of the I Ching.* Aquarian Press, 1989.

Munsterberg, Hugo. *Dictionary of Chinese and Japanese Art.* Hacker Arts, 1981.

Narain, A.K. ed. *Studies in the History of Buddhism.* Dehli: BR Publishing, 1980.

Olschak, B.C. and Wangyai, Thubten. *Mystic Art of Ancient Tibet.* New York, 1973.

Pabongka Rinpoche. *Liberation in the Palm of your Hand.* Ed. Triang Rinpoche. Trans. Michael Richards. Boston: Wisdom, 1991.

Petter, Frank Arjava. *Reiki Fire.* Lotus, 1997.

Picken, Stuart D. B. *Buddhism, Japan's Cultural Identity.* Kodansha.

Pye, Michael. *The Buddha.* Duckworth, 1979.

Rambach, Pierre. *The Art of Japanese Tantrism.* London: MacMillan, 1979.

Rand, Wiliam L. *Reiki, the Healing Touch:* First and Second Degree Manual. Vision, 1991.

Rawson, Philip. *Sacred Tibet.* London: Thames & Hudson, 1991.

Rawson, Philip and Legesa, Laszlo. *Tao.* London: Thames & Hudson, 1973.

Rossbach, Sarah. *Interior Design with Feng Shui.* London: Rider, 1987.

Sangharakshita. *Who is the Buddha?* Windhorse, 1994.

Saso, Michael. *Tantric Art and Meditation.* Honolulu: Tendai Educational Foundation, 1990.

BIBLIOGRAPHY

Saunders, Dale E. *Buddhism in Japan.* University of Pennsylvania UP, 1964.

Saunders, Dale E. *Mudra.* Princeton: Princeton IP.

Saunders, Kenneth J. *Epochs in Buddhist History.* Chicago: University of Chicago Press.

Shimizu, Yoshiaki and Rosenfield, John M. *Masters of Japanese Calligraphy 8th –19th Cenury.* Asia Society of Galleries, 1984.

Simpson, William *The Buddhist Praying Wheel.* New York: University Books, 1970.

Snellgrove, D.L. *Buddhist Himalaya Travel and Studies in the Quest of the Origins and Nature of Tibetan Religion.* Oxford: Bruno Cassirer.

Snellgrove, David. *Indo-Tibetan Buddhism, Volumes I & II.* Shambala, 1987.

Snellgrove, David. *The Images of the Buddha.* Serinda, 1978.

Snelling, John ed. with Mark Watts and Dennis Sibley. *The Early Writings of Alan Watts.* Celestial Arts, 1987.

Society of Chinese Buddhists. *The Sutra of the Lord of Healing.* China, 1936.

Soothill, William Edward and Hodous, Lewis eds. *A Dictionary of Chinese Buddhist Terms.* Dehli: Motilal Banasidoss, 1937.

Soper, Alexander Coburn. *Literary Evidence for Early Buddhist Art in China.* Switzerland: Artibus Asiae.

Stein, Diane. *Essential Reiki: A Complete Guide to an Ancient Healing Art.* Freedom,. CA: Crossing Press. 1995.

Steiniber, Oberlin, E. *The Buddhist Sects of Japan.* George Allen and Unwin, 1938.

Stevens, John. *The Marathon Monks of Mount Hiei.* London: Rider.

Strong, John S. *The Legend of King Asoka–A Study and Translation of Asokávadána.* Princeton: Princeton UP.

Stutley, Margaret and James. *A Dictionary of Hinduism. London*: Routledge and Kegan Paul, 1977.

Talbott, Harold. *Hidden Teachings of Tibet.* London: Wisdom, 1986.

Tansley, David V. *Subtle Body Essence and Shadow.* London: Thames & Hudson, 1992.

Tomio, Shifu Nagaboshi. *The Bodhisattva Warriors.* York Beach, Maine: Weiser.

Tucci, Guiseppe. *The Theory and Practice of the Mandala.* Trans. A.H. Broderick. London: Rider, 1961.

Vaccari, Mrs. and Mr. Oreste. *Standard Kanji.* Tokyo.

Vaswani, T.L. *The Face of Buddha.* India: Cita, 1969.

Vassantara. *Meeting the Buddhas: A Guide to Buddhas, Bodhisattvas and Tantric Dieties.* Scotland: Windhorse.

Waddell, L. Augustine. *The Buddhism of Tibet or Lamaism.* Heffer.

Wayman, Alex. *The Buddhist Tantras.* New York: Weiser, 1973.

Williams, Paul. *Mahayana Buddhism: The Doctrinal Foundations.* London: Routledge, 1989.

Wolf, Fred Alan. *The Dreaming Universe.* New York: Simon & Schuster, 1994.

Yokoi, Yulio. *The Japanese–English Zen Buddhist Dictionary.* Tokyo: Sankibó Buddhist Bookstore, 1991.

Index

INDEX

-Vairocana (see also Dainichi) 17, 18, 23, 40, 61, 64, 130, 143
-Vajradhara 33, 88, 183
-Victorious Healing Tree 95
Buddha Fields 29
Buddha Land (see also Pure Land) 95
Buddha Star System 17
Buddha World 16, 17
Buddhahood 14, 21, 32, 50, 51, 113, 156, 159, 160, 163
Buddhas 32, 74, 114, 125, 175, 178
-Five Dhyani 17, 59, 143
-Five Meditation 51
-Seven Healing 23, 27, 29-31, 34, 43, 88, 184, 195, 197
-Six Healing 16, 47
-Medicine 27
-of the 10 Directions 23, 39, 49, 120, 121
-Fifty Three Past 23, 39, 40
-Seven Male 176, 183
Buddhism
-Tantric 87, 184
-Vajrayana 87
Buddhist
-Shingon 23
-Society of Chinese Buddhists 26
-Tendai 23
-Zen 149, 155, 156
-Monastery 150, 155
-Temple 158
Cady, Duff 5
Celtic Druids 83
Chakras 2, 70, 80, 89, 90, 143
Ch'en, Kenneth 157
Chi 7, 53
Chicago University 19, 147, 149
China 13, 14, 27, 32, 33, 53, 80, 95, 98, 111, 126, 156, 158, 180
-Emperor of 14
Christ, Jesus 2, 25, 140, 153, 154
Christianity 25, 69, 154, 169
Christians 25, 83, 147, 149, 153, 154
Consecrations (see also Initiations) 2, 88, 113
de Visor, J W 180
Dioscuri 42
Direction/s
-Above 13, 16, 39, 140, 180, 181
-Below 13, 16, 39, 140, 180, 181
-Centre 64, 143
-Doorman/Doormen 17, 41, 49, 99, 191
-Eight 16, 33, 80
-Four 13, 41, 44, 50, 52, 143, 191

-Kings of Four 23, 41, 140
-Dhritarashtra 42
-Vaishravana 42
-Virudhaka 42
-Virupaksha 42
-South 13, 14, 15, 39, 44, 52, 61, 68, 83, 100, 121, 177, 180, 191
-Ten 38, 39, 52, 120
-West 13, 15, 21, 39, 41, 44, 52, 62, 68, 79, 83, 121, 143, 177, 180, 191
Distance Healing 37, 72, 90, 137, 193
Dowman, Keith 125, 184
Dreams 55, 56, 183, 192
Earth 12, 18, 26, 29, 80, 83, 117, 128, 140, 175
Earth Mother 31
Elaide, Mircea 70, 148
Elements, Five 13, 17, 18
Endocrine Glands 89
Energy Exchange 151, 168-170
Enlightenment 14, 16, 27, 30, 40, 49, 50, 56, 61, 67, 75, 77, 78, 97, 114, 121, 140, 148, 154, 160, 161, 177, 179, 184, 192
Evil 36, 100
Fairy Tales 20, 148, 152, 164, 172
Feng Shui 13, 45, 47, 49, 50, 158, 180, 187
Five Awarenesses 86, 87
Five Wisdoms 86, 87
God 15, 19, 27, 39, 41, 49, 56, 64, 69, 77, 78, 81, 95-97, 113, 128, 140, 163, 186, 198
-Christian 84
-Jupiter 84
-Indra 83, 181
-Light of 40, 130
-Mithra 98, 157
-Names of 96
-Vrthragna 157
-Zeus 83, 84
-Zurvan 157
Goddesses 33, 34, 68
-Demeter 31
-Eight 191, 192
-Gaia 31
-Great 32
-Great Mother 33
-Hera 31
-Isis 31
-Medicine 31
-Mother 162
-of Earth 32
-sMan-gyi-lHa-mo 31

INDEX

Herbs and other natural health products and information are often available at natural food stores or metaphysical bookstores. If you cannot find what you need locally, you can contact one of the following sources of supply.

Sources of Supply:

The following companies have an extensive selection of useful products and a long track-record of fulfillment. They have natural body care, aromatherapy, flower essences, crystals and tumbled stones, homeopathy, herbal products, vitamins and supplements, videos, books, audio tapes, candles, incense and bulk herbs, teas, massage tools and products and numerous alternative health items across a wide range of categories.

WHOLESALE:

Wholesale suppliers sell to stores and practitioners, not to individual consumers buying for their own personal use. Individual consumers should contact the RETAIL supplier listed below. Wholesale accounts should contact with business name, resale number or practitioner license in order to obtain a wholesale catalog and set up an account.

Lotus Light Enterprises, Inc.

P O Box 1008 RHB
Silver Lake, WI 53170 USA
262 889 8501 (phone)
262 889 8591 (fax)
800 548 3824 (toll free order line)

RETAIL:

Retail suppliers provide products by mail order direct to consumers for their personal use. Stores or practitioners should contact the wholesale supplier listed above.

Internatural

33719 116th Street RHB
Twin Lakes, WI 53181 USA
800 643 4221 (toll free order line)
262 889 8581 office phone
WEB SITE: www.internatural.com

Web site includes an extensive annotated catalog of more than 10,000 products that can be ordered "on line" for your convenience 24 hours a day, 7 days a week.

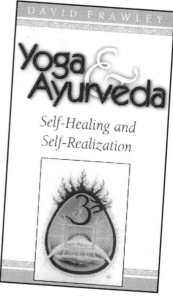

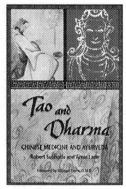

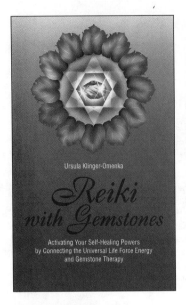

Ursula Klinger-Omenka

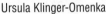

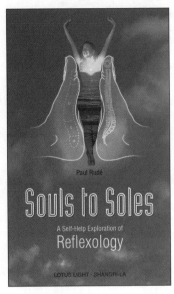

Paul Rudé

Reiki with Gemstones

Activating Your Self-Healing Powers —Connecting the Universal Life Force Energy with Gemstone Therapy

While Reiki, the universal life energy, brings the physical and emotional functions back into their original harmony, gemstones concentrate light-filled powers and color vibrations into the chakras, whose unrestricted functioning is greatly important for vitality and well-being. By connecting Reiki with gemstone therapy, the powers of self-healing are activated in a natural manner. The author writes on the basis of many years of rich experience in working with Reiki and gemstones. She trustingly places her perceptions into the hands of the reader, who can put them to practical use for the good of all beings within a short time.

128 pages, $12.95
ISBN 0-914955-29-2

Souls to Soles

A Self-Help Exploration of Reflexology

Caring for the feet has been part of the culture of many civilizations, for thousands of years. Now bursting forth all over the world, reflexology is being widely accepted as a safe, powerful means of reducing stresses, promoting vitality and well-being.
The author has masterfully captured the essence of reflexology with beautiful illustrations and clearly presented guides for using your touch effectively on the feet. Truly an exploration, this book takes you on a fun loving adventure that has value for all age groups. Breaking new ground, this book also shows you how to reach out to the young, to help them in their times of discomfort, a tender loving experience for those who cannot help themselves.

160 pages, $12.95
ISBN 0-914955-51-9

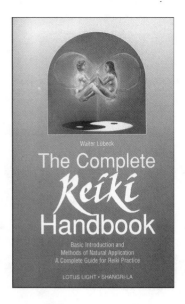

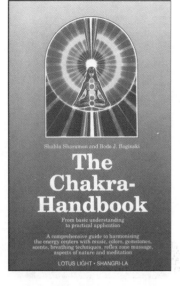

Walter Lübeck

The Complete Reiki Handbook

Basic Introduction and Methods of Natural Application—A Complete Guide for Reiki Practice

This handbook is a complete guide for Reiki practice and a wonderful tool for the necessary adjustment to the changes inherent in a new age. The author's style of natural simplicity, much appreciated by the readers of his many bestselling books, wonderfully complements this basic method for accessing universal life energy. He shares with us, as only a Reiki master can, the personal experience accumulated in his years of practice. Lovely illustrations of the different positions make the information as easily accessible visually as the author's direct and undogmatic style of writing. This work also offers a synthesis of Reiki and many other popular forms of healing.

192 pages, $ 14.95
ISBN 0-941524-87-6

Shalila Sharamon and
Bodo J. Baginski

The Chakra Handbook

From Basic Understanding to Practical Application

Knowledge of the energy centers provides us with deep, comprehensive insight into the effects the subtle powers have on the human organism. This book vividly describes the functioning of the energy centers. For practical work with the chakras this book offers a wealth of possibilities: the use of sounds, colors, gemstones, and fragrances with their own specific effects, augmented by meditation, breathing techniques, foot reflexology massage of the chakra points, and the instilling of universal life energy. The description of nature experiences, yoga practices, and the relationship of each indiviual chakra to the zodiac additionally provides inspiring and valuable insight.

192 pages, $ 14.95
ISBN 0-941524-85-X

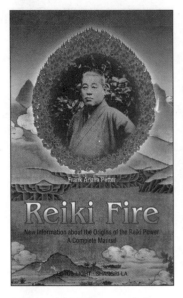

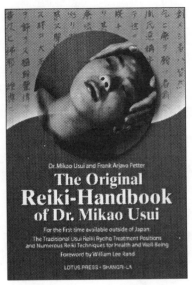

Frank Arjava Petter

Reiki Fire

**New Information about
the Origins of the Reiki Power
A Complete Manual**

The origin of Reiki has come to be surrounded by many stories and myths. The author, an independent Reiki Master practicing in Japan, immerses it in a new light as he traces Usui-san's path back through time with openness and devotion. He meets Usui's descendants and climbs the holy mountain of his enlightenment. Reiki, shaped by Shintoism, is a Buddhist expression of Qigong, whereby Qigong depicts the teaching of life energy in its original sense. An excellent textbook, fresh and rousing in its spiritual perspective, this is an absolutely practical Reiki guide. The heart, the body, the mind, and the esoteric background, are all covered here.

144 pages, $12.95
ISBN 0-914955-50-0

Dr. Mikao Usui and Frank A. Petter

The Original Reiki Handbook

**The Traditional Usui Reiki Ryoho
Treatment Positions and
Numerous Reiki Techniques for
Health and Well-Being**

For the first time available outside of Japan: This book will show you the original hand positions from Dr. Usui's handbook. It has been illustrated with 100 colored photos to make it easier to understand. The hand positions for a great variety of health complaints have been listed in detail, making it a valuable reference work for anyone who practices Reiki. Now that the original handbook has been translated into English, Dr. Usui's hand positions and healing techniques can be studied directly for the first time. Whether you are an initiate or a master, if you practice Reiki you can expand your knowledge dramatically as you follow in the footsteps of a great healer.

80 pages, 100 photos, $ 14.95
ISBN 0-914955-57-8